BODY BALANCE

Vitalize Your Health
with pH Power

KARTA PURKH S. KHALSA, C.D.-N., R.H.

TWIN STREAMS
Kensington Publishing Corp.
http://www.kensingtonbooks.com

TWIN STREAMS BOOKS are published by

Kensington Publishing Corp.
850 Third Avenue
New York, NY 10022

All Kensington titles, imprints, and distributed lines are available at special quantity discounts for bulk purchases for sales promotions, premiums, fund-raising, educational or institutional use.

Special book excerpts or customized printings can also be created to fit specific needs. For details, write or phone the office of the Kensington Special Sales Manager: Kensington Publishing Corp., 850 Third Avenue, New York, NY 10022. Attn. Special Sales Department. Phone: 1-800-221-2647.

ISBN 0-7582-0267-9

First Trade Printing: February 2004
10 9 8 7 6 5 4 3 2 1

Printed in the United States of America

To my teacher and mentor, Yogi Bhajan,
who introduced me to the blessings of natural healing
and who taught me that the greatest motto on earth is "Keep Up!"

CONTENTS

PREFACE

Understanding pH can keep you well. With the knowledge you are about to gain, you can achieve balanced health. And balanced health can be more powerful than disease.

Imagine a time in the near future when you're free from sickness, when you haven't been bothered by even a sniffle or a rash—for years. That future can become a reality.

I'm living proof of the power of natural medicine. I've seen hundreds of patients regain vibrant health, and I'm not alone. An entire new generation of natural medicine therapists is transforming the healthcare system in America. They are using ancient techniques, from around the world, right alongside modern ones. People are listening.

These are hopeful signs at a time when the future of our health is reported to be grim. Amid a rising tide of superbugs and worldwide epidemics, resistant to the best that modern conventional medicine has to offer, in a world where our health professionals themselves admit that disease appears to be outrunning the effectiveness of our medicines, fear is running high among healthcare practitioners and the American public.

I am sure you, like other Americans, want to know what you can do to protect yourself—not only against an unknown future of infectious diseases, but against the degeneration, aging, and daily irritations that undermine the quality of our lives.

A new generation has grown up exposed to natural healing practices. Now that we are really beginning to need them, these techniques are becoming available to everyone. People have never been more concerned about health; about healthcare and its costs, as well as its effectiveness; about the way they fight illness; about the way they age; about the quality of their life. And in an era of rising consumer disenchantment with, suspicion of, and cynicism about conventional Western medicine and its bankrupt paradigms, you probably have never been more interested in what you can do for yourself, by yourself.

At this urgent moment when you and your family are hungry for answers that offer promise, when the superficial treatments on which you have relied are failing you, there is no better investment you can make in your future than to learn and incorporate practical natural health maintenance techniques. In this book, I will make the rich, historically potent traditions of natural healing useful and doable in an everyday way for everyday people.

I am an herbalist, nutritionist, and educator. I have been making natural healing approaches palatable to the modern mind for thirty years. My patients find extraordinary benefits and amnesty from a vast range of health concerns by making these principles part of their lives. For the entirety of that thirty years, I have been a student of an Ayurvedic master, Yogi Bhajan. It has been my good fortune to have been involved in the American renaissance of modern herbalism, and particularly in the introduction of Eastern ideas to Western minds, from the beginning.

For three decades, I have spent my days with sick people in the real world. I have seen what works to confer long-term, vibrant health. I have also seen what does not work. The ideas in this book are not another intellectual theory, but practical, well-developed concepts with roots in ancient traditions and flowers in today's scientific discoveries.

My specialty is making these natural healing concepts understandable by Americans. Most of these ideas are just common sense. If you had grown up in a culture such as China or India, which still has intact natural healing traditions, you would have been introduced to these ideas on your grandparents' knees. Growing up with these concepts and seeing the results all around you makes these concepts natural, not foreign as they are to Americans.

Natural Medicine, Future Medicine

Everyone who is anyone in the health profession today is pointing to natural medicine and self-care as the only doors leading out of the deeply flawed position into which much of our present thinking and our methods and systems of healthcare have confined us.

The practice of acid-alkaline balance, or pH balance, is the ultimate self-care system. Natural healing is all about prevention. The techniques of natural healing and self-care are geared toward keeping you from ever suffering symptoms, and if you do, to bringing you back into balance quickly and effectively so that you don't experience others.

Natural healing has a different vision of the healthy human. A healthy human is not just a gradually failing, getting-through-the-day person, but a vibrant being with energy to excel. In this book, we are going to explore how we can have that type of radiant good health.

Medicine That Americans Can Swallow

In this practical guide to understanding and using natural medicine, we will also take a provocative look at why Americans get sick and stay sick, and how pH balance can keep them well for life. You will welcome—and may even be shocked at—the expanse of knowledge, insight, and often-simple solutions previously unknown to you.

From the unique perspective of a dynamic theory of healing, you will learn how your body works and how it heals. What are the proper foods and herbs to feed your body and why? *Why* can herbs, foods, and spices heal? How do they all fit together? Understanding the body-balance factor will put everything in perspective.

Why *Body Balance?*

I'm sure you've noticed that there are numerous natural healing theories and methods—and that they all seem to conflict with each other. Dr. X tells you to do one thing, while Dr. Y tells you to do exactly the opposite. Presumably, Dr. X and Dr. Y both have had good success with their ideas when they applied them with their patients or they wouldn't be touting them to the public. How could they both be right then?

They can be and they are. This is because no one theory works for everyone. Individualization is the key. We are born into different bodies, each with a different heritage, and we have all lived different lives.

You may have heard of several systems—for example, megavitamins, high-protein diets, high-fiber diets. You may have practiced some. If you got well, you became a convert. If you didn't get well, you went on to the next theory. What we really need is a coherent, systematic way of understanding our individual needs and applying remedies to bring us back to health and happiness in a body that works correctly year after year.

The traditional natural healing systems have already worked out this individualized approach. Any healing system that has been around long enough to study many generations of people has come to the same basic conclusions about how human bodies work. If we dig deep enough, we find them all dipping from the same stream. Only the words are different. Traditional Chinese Medicine and Ayurveda from India, to name the two most well known, are very similar philosophically, but they express their core ideas in different languages and with different cultural concepts. Yet both systems have worked out the idea that people are different and need to be treated differently. And they have worked out techniques to do just that—successfully.

The problem with these systems is that they are huge and complex, great for alternative doctors, but too arcane for the average person. The value of the acid-alkaline-balance perspective lies in its universal application. No matter what your background, there is something you can use from this method. While traditional natural healing systems have contributed immensely to the good of humanity, Body Balance brings in another point of view that will help to fill in the picture of planetary natural healing in the modern world.

In my long search to find a coherent, cohesive theory that explains the success of the spectrum of effective health programs, I have become convinced that the area of acid-alkaline balance deserves serious attention. I want the story to be told. I want basic alternative medicine concepts to make sense to you. I have translated the often-arcane concepts of herbal healing into a language that anyone can understand and appreciate.

Though pH is a concept more modern than those behind the traditional systems, it gives us a measuring tool that people can master and apply. It explains the reason some people get better on one diet and others on other diets. The concept of pH balance is the glue that holds all the various theories, systems, and techniques together. Acid-alkaline balance is one of the least discussed yet most important physiological functions in the body.

Alternative medicine has begun to achieve some degree of recognition in recent years, yet people are still unclear about its basic concepts. Frequently, I speak with persons who have read half a dozen books on complementary techniques and are confused, but still intrigued. Often, after an introduction to acid-alkaline balance, the lightbulb goes on. "This isn't so obscure and metaphysical after all," they say. "I can do this."

A hundred doctors and healers can tell you that natural medicine is the way of the future and they can tell you what to do. You can understand your body, succeed in regaining your health, and develop a personal program that keeps you well. I have done it (and thousands of my patients have as well). You can do it, too. The wealth of information in this book makes sense. I hope it *inspires you to action*.

As we explore together, *Body Balance* will lead you out of the dark about some issues, bust some myths about diet and herbs in general, and present science in everyday language that you can understand. I want to help you pursue optimal health, so that the state of your health can become a source of pleasure and energy instead of a problem. You will be able to make pH-balanced foods and medicinal, healing, nourishing herbs a part of your life, as tonics for better health, energy, stamina, and strength.

Vitamins, specialty foods, and herbs fill the shelves of health food stores. Understanding how to use them for self-care will add a new dimension to your personal health and healing.

You can begin to take steps to live the best life you can live—not only by nourishing your body with a customized, individualized diet based on pH principles, but also by building on that foundation by using herbs, foods, and teas to heal illness, soothe injury, and tip the odds against disease and degeneration in your favor.

The pH perspective can be seamlessly integrated into your life. If you are like the mother who believes that all babies get ear infections; the sinus sufferer who assumes antibiotics and surgery are the only options; the arthritic, the allergic, and the addicted who have been told there is no hope for their conditions, you are in for a great surprise.

Have you ever wondered if your skin rash, hemorrhoids, diarrhea, balding head, and weak eyesight are connected? *Body Balance* will give you the tools to reverse all of these and more with a new perspective on your life. Armed with the knowledge of how you are put together as an individual, you will be able to properly select your diet, understand which herbs to take and what style of massage to have, and even determine at what temperature to keep your office.

Acid-alkaline balancing is systematic and user friendly. You will find the methods in this book easy to understand and logical to apply. As we proceed, acid-alkaline balancing will come through as consistent and eminently useful.

There's much to learn, and it can be easy, fun, and most importantly, effective even beyond what you might imagine. You will become more deeply committed to your health—and you will have powerful new tools with which to do something about it. *Body Balance* will help Americans change the way they see health, disease, medicine, and healing, and will tangibly impact what they can do about it day to day.

The Trip to a Balanced Body

This book is divided into fifteen chapters. Each one will help you as you travel on your journey to understanding and using pH concepts. Along the way, you will reach a new level of health and well-being.

Chapter 1 will introduce you to the body-balance system of natural healing. You'll see why acid-alkaline balance is the most overlooked diagnostic tool in modern medicine. Acid-alkaline balance affects every aspect of health and behavior. We'll look at what pH balance can and can't do, and what new ideas in body chemistry have to offer you.

Chapters 2 and 3 open a door onto the two oldest healing systems on earth: Ayurveda from India and Traditional Chinese Medicine. We will compare ancient ideas about health with newer understanding about chemistry. In Chapter 4, we will explore macrobiotics, a modern adaptation of Asian natural healing principles that has become popular in the United States in the last few decades. Macrobiotic experts have done some interesting work in comparing Asian ideas about physiology with modern pH concepts.

We will talk about practical, everyday uses for these concepts. Chapter 5 will detail sensible applications for using Asian healing concepts and methods in the treatment of disease. We'll meet several practitioners who specialize in using these techniques on a daily basis. In Chapter 6, we'll see how modern naturopathic medicine uses natural healing therapies to balance the body and treat diseases.

Science has uncovered much that is of value to us in our journey to pH balance. We'll look at modern scientific understanding of acid and base in human physiology in Chapter 7. Modern practitioners of alternative medicine apply these body-balancing techniques in practice. In Chapter 8, we'll meet several modern doctors who use these ideas in their practices, and who conduct research on the importance of pH to our overall health. In Chapter 9, we'll explore techniques that physicians use to test acid-alkaline balance. You can use these methods, also. We'll explore several ways you can measure your pH to check on the balance of your body and track your progress toward health.

Chapter 10 delves into food and diet. You will gain insight into how what you eat affects your health and daily performance. We will discuss crafting a diet that will keep you in pH balance and feeling great every day. We will present several delicious recipes that can be a cornerstone of a successful body-balancing program.

Body-balancing techniques can keep all your systems healthy. Chapter 11 will cover the digestive tract, one of the most important systems for balancing your body's pH and maintaining your general health. We will also look at natural treatments for a host of digestive conditions. Since herbal medicine can be a cornerstone of natural treatment, we will go deeply into how you can balance your life and heal your body with pH-balancing herbs. Chapter 12 will give you effective herbal tools to defeat frustrating health problems. In our quest to go even more deeply into lifestyle changes you can use to sharpen your mind and maintain your daily balance, we will cover a selection of home remedies in Chapter 13.

Body balancing can mean the end to suffering from an assortment of bothersome health conditions. In Chapter 14, we will review natural treatments for several ailments and present body-balancing treatments for each. Finally, we all want to live a life of balance. But how can we apply the principles in our daily routine? Chapter 15 goes into detail to help you integrate these diet and herb techniques into your routine to sustain the wonderful changes you can make in the way you live in the world.

How to Use This Book

This book is designed to be used. A good way to approach *Body Balance* is to skim the chapters and get an overview of the territory. Then start at the beginning. For a road map of the subject, see Chapter 1. From there, you can jump first to the chapters that interest you the most.

If natural medicine is your bent, check out Chapters 2 through 6, which detail pH concepts in natural healing systems. If you're inclined toward the scientific approach, you can go straight to Chapters 7 and 8, where we talk about the scientific background and application of these principles. When you are ready to check your personal body-balance status, use Chapter 9 as a guide. There you will find methods you can use immediately to measure your body chemistry.

If you have specific problems, you may want to go straight to the treatment sections in Chapters 12 through 14. You can use these treatments even without the full background of *Body Balance*. For food aficionados, check out the recipes and food ideas in Chapter 10.

Ultimately, no book on health does us any good sitting on the shelf. To feel the tremendous benefits of aligning your personal body chemistry, you have to become engaged and use these techniques. *Body Balance* will be a starting point for your journey to balanced acid-alkaline chemistry, and the great health and stress relief you will achieve with an optimal state of body chemistry.

ACKNOWLEDGMENTS

I wish to thank all those who helped me on my journey through the land of body balancing and natural healing therapy.

Dr. Susan Brown was very helpful in putting together the details of pH and chemistry and in providing leads on the trail of pH studies. My close colleague Dr. Kartar Singh Khalsa showed me how these ideas can affect a person's life for the better. Dr. Michael Tierra, one of the true herbal pioneers in the modern health revival, was full of encouragement and helpful ideas. Dr. Robin Dipasquale, an exceptional physician and herbalist, provided valuable guidance and helped with the naturopathic perspective. Aviva Romm, president of the American Herbalists Guild, was a valuable source of herbal information and insight into women's health issues. Dr. Alan Tillotson, a wealth of herbal knowledge, added valuable details on the Ayurvedic perspective. My longtime colleague Chanchal Cabrera, N.I.M.H., A.H.G., helped with clinical details.

Finally, my wife, Jagdish Kaur, is my partner in everything in life. It was her steady support that allowed me to stay on track and bring this information to the people who will use it.

1

The Body Balance System of Herbal Healthcare

Acid-alkaline balance is the most overlooked diagnostic tool in modern medicine. It has been neglected by modern medical doctors for a century. Like many other seemingly obvious correlations with overall health, pH balance has never become a major area of attention in medical practice. While medical doctors do use measures of pH in specific situations, mainly emergencies, to assess the status of various conditions and tissues, in general they do not routinely monitor acid-alkaline balance.

All living systems depend on proper pH for life. Proper pH goes to the very heart of optimal health in the whole body. Acid-alkaline balance is one of the basic mechanisms, if not the most basic mechanism, of cellular function. Understanding pH will allow all of us to avoid disease, if we use this understanding to help maintain the correct balance. This forgotten knowledge is critical to proper health.

One of the most important aspects of acid and base physiology and their relative concentrations is that they help to maintain a definitive biochemical balance within the body. Through the balance created by the concentrations of these compounds, proper and biologically compatible pH levels are sustained. These levels are very precise and must be carefully guarded and perpetuated in order for cellular function and chemical reactions within the body to occur. Without this delicate balance of pH within the body, life as we know it today would not exist.

If the pH of the body's tissues is off, nothing will function correctly. Every function in the body is dependent on the involved tissues having the proper acidity.

Acid-alkaline balance affects mental functions, mood, and behavior. Alkalinity is a mood elevator. High alkaline producers are peak performers with high lung capacity, good digestive function, and large reservoirs of alkaline minerals in the skeleton.

Robin Dipasquale, N.D., the chairman of the department of botanical medicine at Bastyr University in Seattle, Washington, says that people with sympathetic nervous system dominance have a more acid metabolism, while those with parasympathetic dominance tend toward alkalinity. According to Dr. Dipasquale, our rushed, keyed-up culture is in general too sympathetic. She says, "People who more easily maintain the parasympathetic state are better able to tolerate more acidic foods."[1]

The use of pH measurement as a diagnostic technique can have remarkable benefits. Modern holistic physicians approach the measure of acidity in blood, stool, urine, and saliva in two fundamental ways:

1. The pH of any of the body's fluids (blood, stool, urine, saliva) can be measured individually. The pH of the fluid will reflect the underlying health of the associated organ system. The patient can then be treated with diet and supplements specific to the condition. For example, citric acid (in the form of calcium citrate) can be used to acidify the urine to treat or prevent kidney stones.
2. The pH of all the fluids can be measured and conclusions can be drawn about the patient's overall health. The total metabolism can be treated with foods, herbs, minerals, breathing practices, and lifestyle changes. The pH measurements can then be taken periodically to determine the progress of the overall health improvement.

Over the past century, a body of work on the modern medical understanding of pH balance has emerged. However, while medical doctors understand pH in medical practice terms of cellular and systemic metabolic processes, and understand that it is critical for health at this level, they do not routinely check minor differences in the pH of body fluids or think they are significant.

Yet medical pioneers have gradually begun to experiment and to draw conclusions about the importance of small, but very significant, changes in pH. There is a body of medical information covering the use of acid-alkaline balance. The key is to put all the information together into a meaningful set of tools.

The measurement, understanding, and use of pH is a modern phenomenon, based on the study of chemistry over the last few centuries. Our ancestors did not have the advantage of these modern techniques, but they did have generations of patient observation. By carefully studying generation after generation of patients, they were able to observe certain consistent patterns. They learned, by treating real people, how the individual human body responds to carefully applied food, herbs, and exercise.

Adding the modern concept of acid-alkaline balance to the wealth of natural healing traditions and methods already in our toolbox gives us another powerful flashlight to illuminate the perplexing complexity that is a human being.

The Vocabulary of Natural Healing

It's helpful to have clarity about definitions of terms used frequently to discuss different kinds of medicine. The terms used are sometimes ambiguous, sometimes used interchangeably, and often mean different things to different people.

"Alternative medicine" could include invasive therapies that would not exactly qualify as "natural medicine." These practices are "alternative" not because they are natural or holistic, but because they are outside of the standard medical model.

Personally, I'm not fond of the term "alternative." It suggests a substandard practice, as if a last resort. Just the opposite is true. Much of what the media and the scientific establishment include in the "alternative" definition is perfectly appropriate or even superior as a first choice, especially considering the advantages of the practices. Of course, it goes without saying that natural medicine is far older than modern drug-based medicine.

Modern-day alternative healthcare in North America is a hodgepodge of systems, paradigms, cultures, metaphors, and philosophies. The vocabulary of modern complementary medicine is likewise a sometimes-confusing swamp of archaic terms, foreign names, and modern scientific concepts thrown together helter-skelter. This is a topic of hot debate among contemporary practitioners. Many of the terms that have been in wide use in North American natural medicine for the last century are terms that were common in the 1800s and were used by natural healing practitioners and medical physicians alike; they were part of the medical lexicon of the time. As natural medicine went into decline in the twentieth century, these terms stayed with the system. The medical profession at large went on to develop newer terminology, which was, in turn, adopted by some natural medicine practitioners. Modern practitioners, particularly herbalists, are attempting to reach a consensus on appropriate terminology for the concepts unique to natural medicine. This is not an easy task.

Natural medicine practitioners use some terms to describe physiological processes that are really metaphors for a function that is poorly understood or difficult to explain from a scientific perspective. Many times, the mechanism of action for a given whole herb or food, with its thousands of components, is not known. What can be observed, though, is the clinical response—the action in a real human being in the real world. When all is said and done, natural medicine is being revolutionized in the twenty-first century, and more changes in understanding and nomenclature are sure to come.

"Toxin" is another term that has a variety of meanings. Correctly defined, a toxin is a poisonous chemical that is produced in the metabolism of a life form, such as a plant or an animal. It is usually unstable. When it comes into contact with our tissues, it causes damage. Our bodies often form antibodies to true toxins. In other words, it is a poison produced by a plant or an animal, often bacteria. Bee sting venom contains a toxin. Snake venom contains toxins. Botulism-causing bacteria produce a deadly bacterial toxin. Natural medicine practitioners, however, often use the term to refer to any undesirable materials retained within the body, whether endogenous (produced inside the body) or exogenous (coming from outside the body). These would include residues of cellular processes (such as used-up hormones), synthetic chemicals introduced from the environment (such as dioxin), bodily wastes (such as uric acid), undigested food materials, and of course, conventional toxins (such as snake venom and poisonous mushrooms). The process of detoxification is a very valuable metaphor. Broadly, it just means to get out of the body that which should not be there. Of course, this could mean a lot of different things to a physiologist. Often the mechanism is poorly, or not at all, understood. What we do know, and very well, is that when patients have the symptoms that go along with "retaining undesirable materials" and are "detoxified," they get better.

The various types of medicine are divided up differently, depending on the classification system used. For example, not all naturopathic medicine is herbal medicine, though a specific naturopathic physician may be an herbalist. Not all holistic medicine is naturopathic, though naturopathic physicians are considered holistic health practitioners. Likewise, not all naturopathic medicine is practiced holistically.

"Conventional medicine" is the most common term used to describe the medicine that has evolved in the industrialized West over the past 100 years. Synonyms for this term include "standard medicine" and "orthodox medicine." Some prefer to call this approach "allopathic medicine." (While this paradigm is sometimes called "Western medicine," this definition is not totally precise because Europe is certainly in "the West" and as a whole has a very sophisticated and advanced approach to herbal medicine and natural healing.)

"Allopathic medicine" means "other disease." Originally coined by homeopathic practitioners, the term was used as a way to differentiate homeopathy from "heroic" chemical medicine. The idea was that "allopathic" prescribers use remedies that are "other" than the disease. In other words, they poison or overcome the disease with chemicals that produce rapid and drastic effects. The term was used by homeopathic proponents as a pejorative term for the "scientific" practitioners (those who used drugs and surgery), who eventually evolved into the conventional medical practitioners of today. In many circles, the original derogatory meaning has been lost, and medical doctors sometimes refer to themselves as practicing "allopathic" medicine to distinguish themselves from "natural" prescribers. This term defines a system that uses exclusively drugs and surgical interventions.

"Alternative medicine" is a broad term that covers the gamut of natural and holistic therapies not deemed "conventional." It can also include a host of controversial treatments and therapies that are not necessarily natural, such as unconventional drugs and established drugs used in new ways.

"Holistic medicine" refers to the approach to well-being that emphasizes evaluating and treating the whole body and the whole life of a person, both in sickness and in health. Typically holistic practitioners regard nonnatural therapies as inherently damaging, and prefer natural and nontoxic substances as well as preventive lifestyle measures to promote health. But for the greater "holistic" benefit of the patient's life, they might choose a nonnatural remedy in some cases.

"Natural medicine" refers to the practice of using only substances and techniques that occur in nature, including herbal preparations, vitamins, diet, massage, and exercise.

"Traditional medicine" includes the traditional, usually ancient medical systems of specific cultures, such as Traditional Chinese Medicine (TCM), Ayurveda, and Native American healing. These are all holistic healing systems.

"Herbal medicine" is the art and science of using plants, foods, and spices to maintain health and treat disease. Most of what we know about herbs initially came from their well-developed use in traditional medicine. Herbalism is really a specific modality, or category of treatment, that in traditional systems is used concurrently with lifestyle adjustments, diet, exercise, bodywork, counseling, and other sundry therapies for the body, mind, and spirit. An herbalist may be trained specifically in herbal medicine or may be a health professional with other credentials, such as medical doctor, naturopathic physician, osteopathic physician, homeopathic practitioner, physician's assistant, or nurse practitioner, who studied herbal medicine as well.

"Naturopathic medicine," or "naturopathy," encompasses a combination of modern medicine and traditional healing philosophies and techniques. Naturopathic physicians are general health practitioners trained as specialists in natural medicine, including, but not limited to, herbal medicines. Their training emphasizes natural and holistic approaches, and they are not licensed to prescribe drugs. Naturopathic physicians often choose to specialize in an area of personal interest, so some may use herbs extensively in their practices, while others focus on lifestyle counseling or dietetics. Some naturopathic physicians are advanced herbalists.

"Integrative medicine" as a phrase is becoming increasingly popular as a way to communicate the essence of the approach: combining the best ideas and practices from around the world and from different systems, both conventional and alternative. This approach is also referred to as complementary medicine.

Defining the Territory

Most of the current information and observations about, and awareness of, natural medicine come to us from other societies. On the whole, these societies have much longer histories of experience using these methods, have used them continuously for millennia, give them more credibility, and have persistently developed the art of using them with a complexity that far exceeds any efforts so far made in the United States. Even countries, pretty much solely in Europe, that have aggressively pursued the scientific basis behind natural treatments have taken their cues from established historical use. For example, scientists seeking to investigate which herbs show enough promise to justify the investment of research money start with those herbs that have an ethnobotanical history of particular success.

The majority of other countries, both Western and Eastern, are ahead of America in conceptualizing, understanding, and implementing the use of natural medicine. The East is the source of most of what is known today about herbalism. This knowledge comes collectively from several larger conceptual systems we often hear today called "Eastern healing."

When people use the term "Eastern healing," they usually mean the healing systems of Asia—specifically, those from India, China, Japan, Tibet, and Southeast Asia. Each of these traditional societies has developed distinguishing paradigms about health and healing, but all spring from some essential common ground that we recognize as "Eastern healing," as contrasted to what we call "Western medicine."

In many ways, what is often called "holistic healing" is the next step in the development of healing systems that originated in the East. A primary foundation in the philosophy of those healing systems involves conceptualizing, interacting with, treating, and supporting the whole body, mind, spirit, and social structure of the person, rather than just an ailing or broken part; that is the essence of "holistic" medicine. Holistic medicine also follows its roots in Eastern healing by taking an interest in health rather than disease. Eastern healing is, by nature, holistic.

These medical systems are, of course, founded on much more than just an overall focus on health and the whole person. Each system is also based on experiences and beliefs about the human body and what creates wellness or disease. This worldview provides teachings covering ways to eat, sleep, exercise, and manipulate the influences of diverse internal and external environments. Each paradigm in turn provides tangible tools and conceptual models for applying what you learn in a practical, day-to-day sense.

Energetics

People of ancient cultures experienced the natural world in which they lived, and sought to develop a way to systematically understand their relationship to it. They reasoned that they were made of the same stuff as the rest of the natural world, and were subject to the effects of circumstances in their living environment. In culture after culture, often widely separated by distance and time, people came to remarkably similar conclusions about how their bodies responded to changes in the climate, diet, season of the year, and so forth.

Practitioners in these cultures put together systematic metaphors for how herbs, food, and exercise interact with the body and mind, based on centuries of observation of their patients. Gradually a consensus emerged.

Fundamentally, these experts concluded that "like increases like." In other words, an external factor, when introduced to the body, will create a similar reaction in the body of the person experiencing the change. For example, going out into the cold weather will make the body cold. Eating heavy food will make the body heavy. This seems obvious on the surface, and it is ultimately pretty easy to grasp intuitively, but putting together all the intricacies of every possible effect of every possible herbal medicine on every possible person is a daunting task.

If we think of all the possible effects, such as temperature and moisture, as energies, we can put together a conceptual scheme that explains the complexity of what it is to be a human being but that is consistent and systematic enough for people to learn and apply in daily life. The cumulative effect of these internal and external factors forms a complex metaphor that we call "energetics." This metaphor creates a conceptual model that is intricate enough to represent an entire human being, yet simple enough to be useful.

Energetic evaluation of the body is based on experiencing the body with the human senses. Since everyone experiences the world in subtly different ways, it takes centuries for a consensus to develop among practitioners about any given therapeutic procedure or remedy. Energetics creates a structure in which remedies can easily be identified and understood. According to energetic systems, the sum total of the effect of a diet or supplement is what counts. For example, we may know from modern science that an herb contains antibacterial activity. We want to give that herb to treat an acute bacterial infection. But we also know that the herb tends to increase body temperature—that is, it is "hypermetabolic, or "hot." If the patient has a fever, or is a person who is particularly prone to develop inflammation (heat) that is difficult to control, we would think twice about using that specific herb. It might kill the bacterium very nicely and treat the infection, but the whole person would be worse off as a net total than before we started. Instead, we would seek out an herb that would kill the infection but that has a "cooling" energy. This approach can make a world of difference in clinical practice and gives us an invaluable tool for managing a case for the best in the long term, and for treating the person as a whole human being. We don't want to make people worse while we think they are getting better.

Using an energetic model, we can systematically collate the properties of foods and herbs according to their taste, temperature, effect before and after digestion, and similar factors.

While the modern method of nutrient analysis is to isolate and identify key active ingredients, which is incredibly complicated and far from complete, considering how recent the effort is, the art and science of energetics creates an impression from the whole, allowing us to grasp the overall nature of the remedy and predict with great accuracy the expected consequences of its use.

Using a system of energetics allows the practitioner to match the actions and nature of the medicine to the individual patient. This categorization of the individual by energies is often referred to as "differential diagnosis." This term means something different in energetics than in conventional medicine. Rather than applying this process to diseases, to differentiate one from another and facilitate proper diagnosis, energetic systems apply it to individuals, all of whom might have the same diagnosis in the conventional sense. Line up ten patients with multiple sclerosis or chronic fatigue syndrome or pneumonia and you will find that they all have characteristics in common, but that each case will be as unique as the person manifesting the disease. An herbalist using an energetic paradigm will choose the herbal prescription based on the uniqueness of the case, rather than on the commonality of the medical diagnosis.

The various energetic systems carve up the spectrum of energies in the human body and mind in somewhat different ways. Basically, though, they all look at about the same things. The concepts that are common to just about all systems of herbal energetics are:

- *Temperature*. This implies body temperature, but also is generally construed to mean metabolic rate. The spectrum is from hot to cold.

- *Weight.* This is an observation of body weight and also of the general density of the tissues.
- *Moisture.* This is an observation of the lubricious nature of the body fluids and of the degree of fluid retention.
- *Taste.* This is essentially a measure of the biochemical composition.

Generally speaking, we can divide pH into energetic categories. Acid substances taste hot, and alkaline substances taste cold.

Acid tastes are sour, pungent, and salty. Alkaline tastes are bitter and astringent. Sweet taste is caused from carbohydrates, proteins, and fats, which all produce acid reactions in the body.

Acid-Alkaline Medical Overview

The pH (degree of acidity or alkalinity) of each tissue and organ system in the body must remain within a very narrow range in order for proper biochemical processes to occur. If the acidity of a tissue or the body as a whole drifts outside the proper range, cellular function will diminish and eventually death may occur. Consequently, it is imperative that the body regulate and maintain the varying pH requirements throughout the system in order to function effectively and, more importantly, to survive.

Alan Tillotson, Ph.D., A.H.G., author of *The One Earth Herbal Sourcebook* (Twin Streams, 2001), says, "Acid pH tends to promote inflammation, while excess alkaline pH tends to promote excess mucus. This is especially obvious when we look at the function of the stomach. The acid stomach tends toward burning, while the alkaline stomach tends to fill with mucus, slowing proper digestion."[2]

Susan M. Lark, M.D., one of the foremost authorities in the fields of clinical nutrition and preventive medicine and author of nine books on women's health and healing, points out that the cell, the basic unit of life, has a slightly alkaline pH—on the plus side from 7.3 to 7.4. A proponent of alkalinizing therapies, she reminds us that all our metabolic processes, including our immune systems, digestion, and hormone systems, function best in a slightly alkaline environment.[3]

As a safeguard, the body has any number of intricate and complex systems that carefully monitor pH throughout the body. Further chemical reactions then control any abnormal acid-alkaline deviations. The mechanisms designed to right these fluctuations are known as acid-base buffer systems.

Dr. Lark mentions that a healthy cell contains large amounts of alkaline substances. These include oxygen, bicarbonate, and certain minerals, notably calcium, potassium, and magnesium.[4]

In chemical terms, a buffer is a solution containing two or more chemical compounds that prevents significant variation in pH, regardless of whether additional acid or a base is added to the solution. The buffer systems that are the most active, and therefore the most serious, in the human body are the bicarbonate–carbon dioxide system; the extracellular system, controlled mainly by the concentration of phosphate; and the mineral-rich bone tissue. This elaborate network of powerful chemical buffers is very effective, controlling pH by buffering so tightly that short-term variations in the pH of the significant bodily fluids, especially blood, seldom occur. The body is constantly being flooded with acids created during internal metabolic processes and obtained from outside sources such as acidic foods. It is this continual assault of acids that eventually begins to dampen the efficiency of the physiological buffers, as well as depleting the body of chemicals, including minerals such as calcium that are necessary for correct buffer function.

The body produces acids as a normal part of metabolism. Stress greatly increases this acid load. All muscular movement also increases the production, and therefore the concentration, of the body's metabolic acids. Fats, carbohydrates, and proteins oxidize to produce necessary energy in the body. We couldn't live without them. We burn the energy they create every hour of every day we are alive. But their metabolism again results in acid waste products that must be buffered. The oxidation to produce cellular energy, mostly in the form of body heat, is the largest offender in excess acid production.

In any healthy person, the oxidation and utilization of foods create a wide range of chemicals that immediately impact the acid-base balance (the pH measure of the tissues). When carbohydrates and fats oxidize in the cells, the result is an excessive quantity of carbon dioxide. Carbon dioxide is a toxic waste product, so this substantial production of carbon dioxide is potentially stressful, even toxic, to the whole body. Depending on how efficiently the respiratory system—one way out of the body for waste carbon dioxide—is functioning, a trace amount of carbon dioxide will be exhaled via the lungs. Contrary to what we learned in high school, however, most of the remaining concentration of carbon dioxide does not in fact go out into the air, but combines with water in the body's tissues to produce carbonic acid, pushing the pH of the blood toward the acid range. To prevent this acid from immediately damaging tissues and disrupting cellular processes, the carbonic acid is buffered by alkaline buffering compounds, including, especially, calcium from bone. It is critical that the body maintain the blood acidity in very tight control. The body will draw upon buffering compounds to preserve the proper blood pH to the point of drastically exhausting its reserves. Eventually, through a complex set of metabolic pathways that we will review later, the carbonic acid is finally eliminated through the kidneys.

But if the kidneys are overloaded in their effort to deal with the increased acid load, the blood also becomes stressed attempting to maintain pH balance. These stresses, occurring continually over many years, can create sweeping negative alterations within the body.

All things considered, the average American takes in an excess of acids and acid-forming foods. This excessively acid diet, combined with diminishing tissue reserves of alkaline minerals, results in an acid overburden of the cells throughout the body.

Further complicating the problem is a disproportionate intake of simple sugars, which are decomposed into acid by-products quite rapidly. When the body reaches a point where it is unable to adequately remove these tissue acids, it must transition to storing the acids, and the body will store these acids anywhere it can. If the acidity of the spaces between the cells, one such acid storage dump, rises, cell metabolism, cell respiration, and eventually, cell life and stability are all greatly damaged. It is well documented that enzyme functions are significantly dependent on acid level and temperature in the cell to uphold proper processes. When the pH of a cell is damaged, the normal enzymes in the cell are also negatively affected and the cells may cease to function properly or at all. Sooner or later, if all these changes take place at the cellular level, the cell becomes dysfunctional and the disease process begins.

When the body's pH goes even slightly off, the whole enzyme function of many interconnected systems will also be damaged. These sweeping pH alterations can be seen in the digestive and immune systems and in all the other major life-sustaining systems in the body.

In Dr. Lark's opinion, "If you are taking over-the-counter remedies for stomach upset on a daily basis, you are overly acidic. If you're a chronic allergy sufferer, your alkaline reserves may be strained."

Obviously, a simple, accurate measurement of the body's fluid pH levels can give us valuable information. From these simple measurements, we can infer the acid or alkaline status inside various systems in the body and the degree of physiological stress in different organs and systems. Couple this with other medical information, such as the result of a bone density test, and we have a tool that can help us understand our health in a much deeper way. This approach gives us a coherent way of thinking about body processes in a broad way, and gives us tools to assess progress. Most important, it provides us with a scheme to make consistent changes and to monitor the results, long before we become aware of problems through discomfort or distressing medical tests.

The consensus of virtually all modern holistic practitioners is that the current American diet and lifestyle result in an overly acid condition. Dr. Lark says that "the wear and tear of daily life gradually causes our cells to lose their healthy alkalinity and become more acidic. That makes us more prone to disease. Over 90 percent of Americans become overly acidic during their lifetimes, due in part to their diets."

Therefore, the therapies suggested by these doctors are almost always focused on alkalinizing the metabolism and lean heavily on dietary change and nutritional supplements to adjust the pH in that direction. While it is theoretically possible that any given patient might be tipped toward the alkaline side and could be treated appropriately, the public work of all these clinicians is overwhelmingly centered on educating patients about alkalinizing regimes.

So, what can we do practically to restore the balance? That's what this book is about. A few simple things will go a long way to creating a solid foundation for change. If, as you read on, you suspect you are too acidic, as most Americans are, begin with these initial measures:

- Add alkaline fruits to your diet.
- Add alkaline vegetables (especially green vegetables) to your diet.
- Use green food supplements (especially wheat or barley grass).
- Up your intake of supplemental minerals, including calcium.
- Consider taking sodium bicarbonate and related alkaline substances (such as calcium carbonate).

Energetic models of diagnosis and healthcare are valuable because of their holistic perspective. You don't have to understand modern physiology or chemistry. You need nothing but your senses to perceive the imbalances. If someone is consistently too hot, you can feel that and can deduce possible problems and solutions to those problems according to a systematized understanding. Energetic models draw conclusions about small areas of function from large observable patterns. It helps us see the forest instead of the trees.

Michael Tierra, L.Ac., O.M.D., is one of the forerunners of the North American natural health movement and was one of the first acupuncturists to be licensed in the United States. He is the founder of the American Herbalists Guild and the author of numerous books on health and herbal healing, including *The Way of Herbs* (Pocket Books, 1998) and *The Way of Chinese Herbs* (Pocket Books, 1998). According to Dr. Tierra, pH:

> represents a simplistic Western idea of balance not dissimilar to Chinese Yin and Yang (which is much broader). I think that to be too alkaline, one may be metabolically, what from a traditional Chinese medical perspective, would be equivalent to being too cold. Similarly, to be too acidic would be equivalent to being too hot. However, it is not so simple since an extreme of either may present a deeper level of complication by exhibiting reverse symptoms. Through careful study one would be able to distinguish symptoms between excess or deficient hot or cold. This later level of consideration is usually not considered by Western exponents who are describing alkaline and acid balance in the body. Again it shows a lack of true wisdom to not realize that an extreme of anything will ultimately produce its opposite in a diseased state.

Physiological models, like the study of pH, can also help us draw broad conclusions about the body's internal environment and consequent health status. But they do that by using modern tools of measurement and by putting together small bits of statistical information, like the pH of the stomach contents, urine, blood, and saliva. They draw large conclusions from the accumulation of many measurements. A physiological system can explain, in modern scientific terms, the mechanism for chemical imbalances that create disease. It helps us see the trees that make up the forest.

These two ways of analyzing our health are nicely complementary and form a great two-sided approach to understanding how we function.

2

Ayurveda: Balance in Action

Many of the ideas reflected in *Body Balance* are not new. Ancient peoples realized that to maintain health, balancing the body's functions is crucial. They did not have modern scientific measuring techniques, but they did have their own awareness, sharpened over generations of enduring observations of patients and their problems. With time, they figured out ways of assessing and balancing body chemistry.

One such system is Ayurveda, the holistic healing system of India. Ayurveda says that all disease arises from imbalances in body functions. Of course, Ayurveda has its own way of evaluating and characterizing the balance of the body.

Translated from Sanskrit as "the science of life" (the word comes from *ayus*, which means "life," and *veda*, which means "knowledge," "science"), Ayurveda is a huge collection of interrelated practices that oversee literally every aspect of a person's health and lifestyle. Ancient Ayurvedic adherents observed and experimented with how people could best live to be as happy and healthy as possible. Ayurveda places particular emphasis on the science of longevity, of course focusing on promoting good health throughout that lengthened life. In order to make it to old age in good health, it is important to stay as healthy as possible as the years go by.

Over many generations of patient, careful observation and systematic exploration, Ayurvedic physicians and scholars recorded in encyclopedic writings what they found worked and did not work about every aspect of living. Often they had the opportunity to closely observe the same people over very long periods of time—in extended families over generations, for example. There are libraries in India filled with thousands of years' worth of written records and information in thousands of volumes—all in Sanskrit, of course.

Ayurveda is the oldest continuing healing system on the planet. According to the scholars of Ayurveda, this system is the origin of most healing systems on the planet today; all Asian medical systems evolved from the core of Ayurveda. Even acupuncture, largely thought to be a Chinese modality, may have originated from Ayurveda; archaeological digs in northern India have unearthed accurate acupuncture maps.

Although historians debate the dates surrounding Ayurveda, some authorities maintain that there is evidence of written records for Ayurveda going back 5,000 years and an oral tradition going back thousands of years before that. Ayurveda offers the layperson a framework for understanding the body and how to best support its quest for balance.

Ayurvedic Energetics

Ayurveda is a complete approach to health and lifestyle management. The system incorporates diet, exercise, life activity routines, psychotherapeutic practices, massage, and of course, botanical medicine, which is the foundation of Ayurvedic therapeutics.

Therapy in Ayurveda is based on an understanding of the underlying concepts of energetics inherent in the Ayurvedic worldview. Ayurveda assigns all matter-energy interactions in the world to a scheme of five primal elements: earth, water, fire, air, and ether. These primal elements, called *mahabhuta* in Sanskrit, are metaphorical concepts that describe physiological processes and environmental interactions. Earth represents the principle of inertia. Water represents the principle of cohesion. Fire represents the principle of radiance. Air represents the principle of vibration. Ether represents the principle of pervasiveness.

The five primal elements are not elements in the conventional sense. They are not substances like hydrogen and carbon. Rather, they are cosmic principles, or prototypes, that provide the basis for the creation of grosser materials. We could call them states of existence. They represent an energy spectrum—a continuum from gross energy to more subtle energy. Ayurveda divides up all the possible matter and energy interactions in the universe into these five categories as a way to conceptually capture all the ways energy can behave. All matter, including our bodies and the environment in which our bodies function, arises out of combinations of these primal energies.

In our bodies and in the universe, all phenomena are created from the five elements. Furthermore, according to Ayurveda, like increases like. If you are already hot and you are exposed to more heat (fire element)—say, by going outside in the summer—you will get hotter. If you are heavy and you eat ice cream, which is also heavy (earth element), you will get heavier. Ayurveda uses this principle of "like increases like" to bring about balance. Since eating a cucumber is cooling (water element), we can use this principle to cool down a condition that is too hot, such as skin inflammation. For the nature, qualities, and effects of the five elements, see Table 2.1.

For ease of conceptualizing the actions of these energies and for therapeutic application in diagnosis and treatment, the five elements, as they manifest in the body, are further condensed into three primal metabolic forces called *doshas*. These metabolic forces underlie all of the theoretical foundation of Ayurvedic diagnosis and therapeutics.

The doshas are responsible for promoting and sustaining balance in the daily and lifelong health of the individual. Ayurveda defines disease as an imbalance in the doshas.

The doshas are characterized by the energies intrinsic to each of these "master forces." These traits include factors such as temperature, moisture, weight, and texture. (See Table 2.2.)

Kapha dosha maintains structure, solidity, and lubrication in the body, forming connective and musculoskeletal tissues. It is wet/oily, cold, heavy, slow, and stable, and in the body it manifests those qualities. It is *anabolic* (tissue building) in function. This energy predominates in the chest and stomach. These are the areas where mucus concentrates are the most alkaline. Dr. Tillotson confirms this when he says, "Asthma patients, in particular, tend to be overalkaline."

Pitta dosha maintains the digestive and glandular secretions, body heat, and metabolism, including the digestive enzymes and bile. It is wet/oily, hot, light, and intense. It is *metabolic* (tissue fueling) in function. Pitta predominates in the small intestine, the most intense region in the body, with the highest metabolic rate. Generally, we can say that pitta correlates with acidity (the Ayurvedic metaphor is "fire"). This really describes intensity, however. It is a metaphor for destruction, especially the destruction of the digestive process. Ayurveda says that bile is the most concentrated essence of pitta. Of course, the bile is the most al-

Table 2.1. The Characteristics of the Five Elements					
	Earth (Solid)	Water (Liquid)	Fire (Power)	Air (Gas)	Ether (Space)
Nature	Fixed, rigid (Substance with stability)	Flux (Substance without stability)	Transforming (Form without substance)	Mobile, dynamic (Existence without form)	Vacuum (Distance without physical existence)
Qualities	Heavy, rough, hard, slow, stable, gross, tough, dry, dense, smelly	Liquid, oily, cold, slow, soft, smooth, dull, slimy, strong taste	Hot, intense, subtle, light, dry, clear, sharp, oily, vision promoting	Light, dry, cold, rough, clear, subtle, soft, oily, touch promoting	Soft, light, subtle, smooth, sound promoting
Pharmacological effects	Plumpness, heaviness, compactness, stability	Stickiness, oiliness, compactness, softness, moisture, contentment	Heat, oxidation, metabolism, luster, radiance, color	Roughness, dryness, lightness, aversion	Softness, porosity, lightness
Sense and organ	Smell Nose	Taste Tongue	Vision Eye	Touch Skin	Hearing Ear
Action and organ	Excretion Anus	Procreation Genitals	Walking Feet	Holding Hand	Speech Mouth
Positive effect	Stability	Juiciness	Clarity	Vigor	Illumination of silent mind
Negative effect	Petrification	Stickiness	Manipulation	Exhaustion	Ache of hollowness

Table 2.2. The Characteristics of the Doshas			
	Kapha	**Pitta**	**Vata**
Elements	Earth and water	Water and fire	Air and ether
Function	Solidity, stability, lubrication, tissue building	Digestion, metabolism, assimilation, body heat, glandular secretion	Movement, nerve regulation, respiration, circulation, excretion
Moisture	Oily (wet)	Oily (wet)	Dry
Temperature	Cold	Hot	Cold
Density	Heavy	Light	Light
Viscosity	Viscous, dense	Fluid	Mobile, rarified
Action tendency	Stable	Intense	Irregular
Texture	Smooth	Liquid, malodorous	Rough
Energy state	Potential	Balancing	Kinetic
Regulates (physical)	Stability, energy, lubrication, slipperiness	Body heat, temperature, digestion, hunger, thirst	Movement, breathing, natural urges, tissue transformation, motor and sensory functions
Produces (emotional)	Forgiveness, greed, attachment, possessiveness	Perception, understanding	Spaciness, fear
Initiates disease process	5% of people	15% of people	80% of people

kaline fluid in the body. The stomach acid is also a site of pitta and is probably the most acid fluid in the body.

Vata dosha maintains movement in the body, such as respiration and joint mobility. It is dry, cold, light, and irregular. It is *catabolic* (eliminative) in function. Vata predominates in the large intestine. The fecal contents are supposed to be slightly acidic, but generally we can consider the effect of cooling vata throughout the body to be slightly alkaline.

From the Ayurvedic point of view, all functions occurring in the body at any one moment are a result of the doshas. Every single action affects their balance. The three doshas are ebbing or flowing in the body at any given time.

Ayurvedic Energetics and Food

Ayurvedic therapeutics is also based on the concept of the five primal elements, or states of existence. The five elements form the foundation of the theories of anatomy, physiopathology, and pharmacology. Ayurveda considers it necessary to know only the state of proportionate balance of the elements in all the parts of the body to shape an accurate diagnosis. Ayurveda does name diseases, but only for the convenience of discussion; diagnoses are based on the energetics of the individual cases.

As the body is composed of the five elements, so are all the other substances on the planet likewise composed. Nutritional and botanical medicines interact with the tissues of the body according to the innate characteristics of their five-element profile.

Foods and herbs are classified as to pharmacology based on several factors: taste (biochemical composition), qualities (physiological action), potency (effect on metabolic rate), and post-digestive effect. Historically, the major systems of natural medicine, including Ayurveda, also organize the clinical actions of foods and herbs according to the energetic property of temperature.

Temperature

Temperature, called *Virya* in Sanskrit, is probably the most basic and significant type of energy in a food or herb. The categorization of temperature is subjective and based on qualities in the patient's reaction to the substance. (See Table 2.3.)

	Heating Herbs (Basically Acid)	Cooling Herbs (Basically Alkaline)
Examples	Mustard, clove	Dandelion, sandalwood oil
Actions	Increase circulation, increase appetite, raise body temperature	Slow down the metabolism, reduce inflammation, treat fever
Promote	Digestion, dizziness, thirst, fatigue, sweating, burning sensations	Refreshing feeling, tissue firmness, calm, clarity
Dosha effects	Increase pitta, decrease kapha and vata	Decrease pitta, increase kapha and vata

Table 2.3. The Characteristics of Herbs

Ayurveda has only two temperature classifications: cold and hot. For example, salad vegetables are cold, while garlic is hot.

Hot characteristics in foods and herbs increase metabolic rate and open circulation throughout the body. Body temperature goes up, but that's not all. Chemical reactions of metabolism go faster. We burn more nutrients. We can actually lose body fat as these nutrients are burned and the temperature of the body goes up, a function called *thermogenesis.* The more nutrients we burn, the more acids we produce that have to be chemically neutralized in the body. Heat is the most basic property of inflammation. Hot substances are pro-inflammatory over time. Since heat burns up tissues, it is considered catabolic.

We all know what happens when we fill up on too much salsa. We get hot, we sweat, and our capillaries expand to allow an increased blood flow, giving us that red face. Hot temperature could be called "hypermetabolic."

Cold temperature might be a little trickier to grasp. Cold herbs slow down metabolic rate and suppress circulation. Body temperature goes down. We literally tolerate cold temperature poorly. Metabolic reactions slow down. We conserve nutrients, or fail to metabolize them in the digestive tract. Cold substances generally make people fatter. Because cold suppresses metabolism, we burn fewer nutrients and liberate less acid, so the body has less acid stress to neutralize. On the other hand, if the body is too cold, it can't properly eliminate waste through blood circulation. It can't burn nutrients to run essential functions.

Celery juice is a good example of a cold food. Even if you consume it at room temperature, you feel yourself getting cooler. Celery reduces inflammation. In fact, it's a great treatment for allergies. Celery slows you down and puts you to sleep. Cold temperature could be called "hypometabolic."

Of course, there are degrees of effect. An herb like cayenne is probably the hottest substance anyone is likely to come across, while cucumber is considered a very cooling food. In Ayurveda, people learn these distinctions from experience.

Temperature is a complicated issue, involving many chemical factors, but essentially we can say that acid creates heat and alkaline promotes cold. Other factors not related to pH come into play when considering the action of temperature. Remember, however, that Ayurveda seeks balance, so neither temperature is superior.

Taste

In Sanskrit, the word for taste, *rasa*, has many meanings. The interrelated nature of the definitions helps us conceptualize the importance of taste in Ayurveda. *Rasa* means "essence," a window into the Ayurvedic idea that taste is perhaps the key factor in understanding the qualities of a plant. *Rasa* also means "sap," a metaphor for the taste of an herb reflecting the qualities of the sap that nourishes the medicine when it is growing. In addition, *rasa* can mean "appreciation," "artistic delight," or a "musical note," all reflecting the same basic idea.

Ayurveda says that taste directly affects our nervous system through the *prana*, the life force. Taste stimulates the nerves, the mind, and the senses; it makes us lively. Through stimulating the gastric nerves, taste enhances digestion.

Ayurveda predicts the physiological effect of a food or medicine by its intrinsic biochemical makeup, which can be identified by taste. Ayurveda recognizes six tastes: sweet, sour, salty, pungent, bitter, and astringent. (See Table 2.4.)

Sweet-tasting plants' active compounds are often carbohydrates or amino acids (proteins). These foods are builders, promoting tissue mass and health. They are the macronutrients. Sweet-tasting plants form the bulk of most diets around the globe. All grains and nuts are predomi-

	Sweet (Produces acid by-products)	Sour (Acid)	Salty (Acid, occasionally alkaline)	Pungent (Acid)	Bitter (Alkaline)	Astringent (Alkaline)
Table 2.4. The Six Tastes						
Elements	Earth and water	Earth and fire	Water and fire	Fire and air	Air and ether	Air and earth
Composition	Carbohydrates, proteins, fats	Organic acids	Minerals (alkalis)	Capsaicin and similar	Alkaloids and other principles	Polyphenols (tannins)
Characteristics	Pleasing, brain tonifying, anabolic	Digestive, sialagogus, anabolic	Moistening, expectorant, anabolic	Detoxifying, cardiac, catabolic	Appetizing, drying, cooling, catabolic	Stiffening, absorbent, catabolic
Temperature	Least cold	Medium hot	Least hot	Hottest	Coldest	Medium cold
Postdigestive effect (vipak)	Sweet	Sweet	Sour	Pungent	Pungent	Pungent
Moisture	Wettest	Least wet	Medium wet	Driest	Medium dry	Least dry
Weight	Heaviest	Lighest	Medium heavy	Medium light	Lightest	Least heavy
Food examples	Wheat, rice, milk, sugar, dates, licorice, peppermint	Yogurt, cheese, green grapes, lemon, hibiscus, rose hips, tamarind	Salt, kelp	Onion, chiles, ginger, garlic, radish	Turmeric, rhubarb, fenugreek, dandelion root and leaves	Unripe banana, pomegranate, goldenseal root, alum

Table 2.4. The Six Tastes (continued)						
	Sweet (Produces acid by-products)	Sour (Acid)	Salty (Acid, occasionally alkaline)	Pungent (Acid)	Bitter (Alkaline)	Astringent (Alkaline)
Actions (cont'd.)	Increases rasa (juiciness), water, ojas, strength; relieves thirst; creates burning sensation; nourishes and soothes, cools	Stimulates appetite, sharpens mind, strengthens sense organs, causes secretions and salivation	Promotes digestion and salivation, acts as antispasmodic and laxative, nullifies other tastes, causes water retention	Cleans mouth, promotes digestion and absorption of food, purifies blood, cures skin disease, reduces blood clots	Promotes other tastes, acts as antitoxic and germicidal, serves as antidote for fainting, treats itching and burning sensations	Sedates, constipates, constricts blood vessels, causes coagulation of blood
Dosha effects	Decreases vata and pitta, increases kapha	Decreases vata, increases pitta and kapha	Decreases vata, increases pitta and kapha	Decreases kapha, increases vata and pitta	Decreases pitta and kapha, increases vata	Decreases pitta and kapha, increases vata
Disorders produced	Obesity, excess sleep, heaviness, lethargy, loss of appetite, cough, diabetes, abnormal growth of tissue and muscles	Increased thirst, teeth sensitivity, eye closure, liquefaction of kapha, blood toxicity, edema, ulceration, heartburn, acidity	Blood disorders, heat disorders, fainting, skin diseases, inflammation, digestive ulcer, rash, pimples, hypertension	Heat, sweating, fainting, burning sensation in throat and stomach, heartburn, digestive ulcer, dizziness, unconsciousness	Roughness, emacination, dryness, reduced bone marrow and semen, dizziness, unconsciousness	Dry mouth, distension, constipation, speech obstruction, heart disorders

Table 2.4. The Six Tastes (continued)						
	Sweet (Produces acid by-products)	Sour (Acid)	Salty (Acid, occasionally alkaline)	Pungent (Acid)	Bitter (Alkaline)	Astringent (Alkaline)
Tissue effect	Anabolic	Anabolic	Anabolic	Catabolic	Catabolic	Catabolic
Emotion	Satisfaction	Envy	Enthusiasm	Extroversion, anger	Dissatisfaction	Introversion

nantly sweet. The root of asparagus is a sweet herb that is used for kidney and lung problems. Most general long-term nourishing tonics are sweet; research is revealing that many immunostimulant tonics have in common a certain kind of long-chain carbohydrate called *polysaccharides*. Carbohydrates, proteins, and fats all potentially increase acidity in the body and must be balanced by other, more potent tastes, those contained in the micronutrients.

Foods with a sour taste produce their action through organic acids. Sour foods cleanse the body of toxins and promote digestion. Acidic foods tend to be high in vitamin content; for example, lemons are high in vitamin C. Citrus peels are, in fact, used herbally to promote digestion and stimulate appetite. Rose hips are sour therapy, contain vitamin C, and are used for the respiratory tract. Sour taste is acid by definition.

Salts are mineral compounds that help the body retain fluids and improve digestion and bowel action. Salty foods and herbs, such as kelp, act to control gas and are given for coughs. Salty taste usually comes from sodium chloride (table salt). This chemical is necessary for nutrition, but contributes to the acid load. Other minerals, less abundant in our diet, also usually have a salty taste. Some, like calcium, have a vaguely salty taste, but are alkalinizing.

Substances with "bite," or pungent herbs, increase digestive secretions. These foods usually contain volatile oils—ginger, for example. Black pepper is an excellent pungent medicine and is used in Ayurvedic therapy as a digestive tonic and blood purifier. Asafoetida, or hing, from the carrot family, is a gum resin from the rootstock of an Asian plant.

With a strong characteristic odor, hing can be used for increasing glandular secretions, enhancing circulation, and rebuilding nerve tissue. Other pungent foods found in the well-known fennel family include dill, coriander, caraway, cumin, and anise, which are all excellent digestive and antiflatulence (carminative) remedies. The "herbs of life," as my mentor, Yogi Bhajan, terms them, include pungent marjoram, rosemary, oregano, and thyme. These pungent foods heat up the body and are basically acidic.

Bitter foods and herbal preparations often contain alkaloids and glycosides as components. Polyphenols, including those found in grapes and green tea, also often contribute to bitter taste. Leafy greens are mildly bitter. These medicines are cleansing and can remove toxins from the tissues. Many pharmaceutical drugs that have been created from plants, such as digitalis from foxglove, come from this bitter category. The king of the bitter herbs is turmeric (the herb that gives the yellow color to curry). Turmeric has wide use in Ayurveda, from treatment of stomach ulcer when mixed with parsley to use for arthritic joints when mixed with milk and almond oil. Bitters can help to balance a rich diet high in sweets and fats. Bitter-tasting foods are alkalinizing.

Astringency, the taste produced by the presence of chemical constituents called tannins, a subcategory of polyphenols, is characteristic of those herbs and foods that are used to promote tissue contraction and fluid absorption. They are used in the treatment of diarrhea, hemorrhage, or excessive urination. The astringent (tightening, drawing) leaves of strawberry, raspberry, and blackberry are used as toning herbs for the mucous membrane of the digestive tract, the uterus, and the kidneys. Plant gum resins—for example, frankincense, myrrh, and gum benzoin—treat by drying areas such as skin and sites of inflammation.

Since most Americans are too acid in pH, the most common recommendation is to concentrate on increasing bitter and astringent tastes.

Ayurveda divides all energies into pairs—cold and hot, for example. Since there are six tastes, with a gradation of effects, the energy pair is expressed as a spectrum. For temperature, the gradations are most hot, medium hot, least hot, least cold, medium cold, and most cold. For weight, they are heaviest, medium heavy, least heavy, least light, medium light, and lightest.

Constitution

The exceptional system of Ayurvedic body typing is also based on the characterization of the three doshas—the three "primal metabolic forces."

In a human body, the predominant dosha, the one most likely to overpower the other two, defines that person's "constitution," or body type. Therefore, the doshas—kapha, pitta, and vata—not only represent specific symptom and disease tendencies, or "leanings" (such as hot or cool, dry or moist), they also identify the body types that manifest those doshas. For example, pitta, as the name of a "master force," refers to a specific set of energy properties or symptoms, but is also the name of a constitutional body type—one in which the body is most likely to demonstrate pitta-type strengths, deficiencies, and inclinations. The pitta body type—the type in which pitta predominates—will be most likely to overemphasize pitta trends and tendencies and to develop an overabundance of pitta, resulting in typical pitta diseases.

Doshas are often thought of as faults, since they represent the ways in which a particular type of energy tends to go out of balance. They are "master tendencies" that can go out of whack in the body at any given time, if allowed to do so. Each dosha tries to overwhelm the other two and dominate. The other two fight back and try to restore equilibrium. You can think of the doshas like the three legs of a stool: one leg always wants to get longer than the others and tip the stool. The job of the other two then is to stretch out and help the stool regain balance.

The fundamental concerns, therefore, when looking at health from an Ayurvedic approach are:

- The relative balance of the doshas at a given moment and the short-term issue of symptoms and disease
- The *constitution*, defined by our primary dosha, and the long-term issue of what it will tend to do over the rest of our lives

This system of understanding your body and mind is incredibly valuable because it is an excellent predictor of how your body will grow and change over the course of your lifetime. When you can predict with great accuracy the types of diseases to which you are most susceptible, you can act well in advance to prevent them. Ayurveda lets you develop preventive living. Your constitution establishes the long-term likelihood for your body to slip into ill health in very particular ways. By understanding those ways, you can live in ways that prevent problems and draw the most on your inherent gifts.

Similarly, the pH perspective gives us an idea of whether our genetic heritage inclines each of us toward being "constitutionally" acid or "constitutionally" alkaline.

Determining Your Body Type

Ayurvedists teach that the constitution is already determined by the time birth occurs. Characteristics of a particular constitution are evident in infancy.

In most Americans, all three doshas have become totally wacky by adulthood, largely due to the way we live and care for ourselves. Children who grow up in surroundings that are adjusted to harmonize their constitutions will consistently display classic signs of their body types throughout life. For many Americans, though, trying to recognize which dosha primarily drives their health is puzzling because so much of what seems to be a big and permanent issue is actually the result of an early and ongoing lifestyle imbalance. In a society marked by unhealthy eating, smoking, drinking, drug abuse, and sedentary lifestyle, this is not surprising. For a general constitutional overview of the three doshas, see Table 2.5.

There are endless possible body types because not all bodies manifest the tendencies of one primary dosha. There are dual-dosha types and even a tri-dosha type in which all three—vata, pitta, and kapha—are about equally strong. Likewise, your constitution can be anywhere on the pH spectrum, from extremely alkaline to neutral to extremely acidic.

For convenience, Ayurveda commonly divides body types into seven categories:

1. Vata (alkaline)
2. Vata-pitta (moderately acid)
3. Pitta (acid)
4. Pitta-kapha (moderately acid)
5. Kapha (alkaline)
6. Vata-kapha (alkaline)
7. Tri-dosha (neutral)

	Kapha (Alkaline/Wet)	Pitta (Acid)	Vata (Alkaline/Dry)
Location (primary concentration of dosha/main problem area)	Chest and stomach	Small intestine	Large intestine
General nature	Solid, smooth, slow, lethargic, slimy	Intense, aggressive, athletic, a leader	Variable, weak, frail
Temperature	Cold	Hot	Cold
Moisture	Oily (wet)	Oily (wet)	Dry
Frame	Thick, large, no definition	Medium, pronounced muscle definition	Slender, tall or short, disproportionate, visible veins and tendons
Weight	Heavy, obese	Moderate	Low
Skin	Thick, oily, cool, pale	Red or yellow, moles, freckles, rashes, warm, soft, prone to perspiring	Rough, dry, cool, dark
Hair	Thick, dark	Scanty or bald, gray or red	Dry, kinky
Appetite	Regular, steady, slow to hunger (hyperglycemic)	Sharp, large	Variable, generally low, needs frequent meals (hypoglycemic)
Digestion	Smooth, efficient	Rapid, hot, acid	Irregular, prone to gas
Feces	Coated with mucus, thick, heavy, regular to slow bowel habits	Oily, burning, prone to diarrhea	Dry, hard, prone to constipation

Table 2.5. Constitutional Overview

Table 2.5. Constitutional Overview (Continued)		
	Kapha (Alkaline/Wet)	**Pitta (Acid)**	**Vata (Alkaline/Dry)**
Mental	Well-considered conclusions, placid, calm, receptive	High intelligence, sharp, irritable	Fluctuating, moody, euphoric, relentless, curious
Memory	Prolonged	Good	Generally poor—good in the short term, but poor in the long term
Emotional strengths	Loyal, calm, stable	Productive, intelligent, determined	Creative, artistic
Emotional weakness	Depression, greed, attachment problems	Jealousy, aggression, judgmental	Anxiety, fear, insecurity
Sleep	Prolonged, deep	Sound	Insomnia, erratic
Dreams	Water, romance	Fiery, passionate	Flying, jumping, running, tall things
Habits	Regular, considered, water	Volatile, foolish, hunting	Hasty, erratic, moving, traveling
Profession	Business, cosmetics	Sports, politics	Drama, dance
Activity	Slow	Athletic	Restless
Menstruation	Easy, regular, light bleeding, prone to edema	Regular, profuse bleeding, bright red blood, prone to premenstrual syndrome and moderate cramps	Irregular, missed, scanty, dark blood, prone to cramps
Sexual	Strong, sensual, low but constant libido, devoted, high fertility	Moderate libido, passionate, domineering, moderate fertility	Variable, low libido, deviant, prone to fantasizing, strong desire, low energy, low fertility

Table 2.5. Constitutional Overview (Continued)			
	Kapha (Alkaline/Wet)	**Pitta (Acid)**	**Vata (Alkaline/Dry)**
Disease tendencies	Mucus, strong immune system, sinus/respiratory problems, kidney problems/edema, tumors abnormal growth or secretion	Inflammation, hypertension, fever, liver problems, acid, skin problems, hemorrhoids, irritable bowel syndrome, rheumatoid arthritis	Pain (all types), headache, osteoarthritis

Fortunately, there is no "best" body type to be. Each has its advantages and disadvantages, its strengths and weaknesses. Single-dosha constitutions tend to have fewer total problems, but the ones they have tend to be more serious. Dual-dosha types and the tri-dosha type tend to have a wider variety of less severe problems.

The constitution verifies not only characteristics of the body. The mind, of course, is also a part of the whole person. The constitution predicts personality characteristics.

The fire type, pitta, tends to be, well, fiery! Pitta personalities are likely to be leaders, passionate, colorful, argumentative, competitive, decisive, and convincing. The air type, vata, is the creative, nervous type. These people are restless and disorganized (in other words, "spacey"). The kapha type is destined to be (what else?) down-to-earth: conservative, loyal, slow, calm, and steady. The very descriptions—earth, air, and fire—evoke pictures that influence our perceptions of people to a large extent.

On the planet as a whole, there is thought to be roughly an equal number of the constitutional categories present in the population.

Pitta constitution is the stereotype of an acidic constitution, while kapha and vata are essentially alkaline constitutional types, with kapha being wet and vata dry.

Working with Your Constitution

Ayurveda uses foods, teas, herbs, and nutrient substances to enhance your gifts—those aspects of your constitution that are advantages. You can also offset your constitution's potential downside. At any given time, you can eat, supplement, or follow some other lifestyle practice to address a specific, current issue of balance. Concurrently, you can also do things that enhance the benefits of your long-term constitution and that ease and soothe the natural tendencies of the body you inherited in order to stave off health problems of the future.

When you have one dosha that is clearly dominant, your entire health-maintenance scheme is concentrated on suppressing that one dosha. If you are vata constitution, then vata is what wants to get inflated in comparison to the other two and bring you out of balance; your vata tendencies will cause certain fundamental vulnerabilities to flare up or show themselves as symptoms. Thus, your efforts—the way you eat, exercise, supplement, and live—should be angled toward keeping vata under control.

Balance can be achieved by strengthening the other two, nondominant doshas, in effect raising their profiles, which is conceptually the same as working to suppress or calm the dominant one.

In a tri-dosha person, all three "master forces" are trying to conquer the other two, vying for the number-one position. Balancing this body type can be challenging; the strategy is like a tightrope balancing act.

Constitutional Healing

Ayurvedic herbal medicine begins by addressing the current collection of symptoms, which may reflect an imbalance of any proportion of the doshas. It then works with the true constitution. To begin with, a body may be very much out of balance, and the symptoms may not be symptoms that are normally associated with the body's constitution type.

Even when you are generally balanced and healthy, conditions may crop up that are representative of any dosha. "Treating pitta" doesn't always mean treating a person with a pitta constitution. It may mean treating a pitta condition in *any* person. For example, a kapha-constitution person with a fever (a pitta condition of excess heat) will need an antipitta remedy temporarily, though that person may return to antikapha treatment for the long-term management of the constitution.

Any person may display symptoms at any time in his or her life that are not typical of the core body type. This reflects imbalance or illness. For example, a pitta-constitution person can certainly experience symptoms involving cold and mucus; these are symptoms of a kapha imbalance and indicate that kapha must be treated. A kapha-constitution person can experience rough, hoarse, dry symptoms; vata is out of balance and must be treated. Once the body is healthy and these circumstances have been dealt with, however, the core conditions that the person will most likely have to deal with throughout life will be those emblematic of his constitution. Once layers of symptomatic imbalances that obscure the true constitution are cleared out, the goal is to head off the most predictable dysfunctions.

The goal of the body-typing system is not to pigeonhole yourself or paint yourself into a corner. That would be the antithesis of Ayurveda. The idea is to note your potential issues and live your life consciously, with awareness.

Personalizing Your Diet with Ayurveda

Each of us is unique. As individual as our body type is, so, too, are our nutritional requirements. Ayurveda recognizes this and emphasizes the correct diet for each individual.

Diet is the first and most basic building block of good health in Ayurveda and can be an effective treatment for disease, even when used alone. It is the safest therapy and can be used by anyone as self-care. Of course, the results may materialize more slowly than with more directed methods, such as herbal medicine.

Improper diet is the main underlying physical factor that induces disease. So, when we modify the diet, we also get at one of the underlying problems.

Ayurveda primarily evaluates the diet based on the energetic qualities of the foods and their effects on the doshas, not necessarily on the chemical (nutrient) content.

Diets for the Doshas

To achieve balance, the diet should have the characteristics that are opposite those of the dosha that is dominating and causing the problem. Kapha is cold, wet, and heavy. Therefore, a diet to control kapha and bring the body to overall balance would emphasize warm, dry, and light foods. Since the main feature that distinguishes kapha is heaviness, focus especially on light (low-fat, easy-to-digest) food.

Pitta dosha is hot, wet, and light. To balance pitta throughout the body, eat a diet that is generally cooling, drying, and grounding. Since pitta is the hot dosha, focus primarily on foods that cool the body.

Vata is cold, dry, and light. To balance vata, follow a dietary program that is warm, moisturizing, and heavy. This type of diet promotes tissue building.

Taste Proportions

When you are treating a dosha that is in excess, you can adjust the proportion of each taste in the diet to balance the body's energetics.

Remember, vata is the dosha that causes frailty, weight loss, and instability. To treat vata, emphasize the anabolic tastes—sweet, sour, and salty. Limit your use of the catabolic tastes—pungent, bitter, and astringent. Salty is best because it promotes water retention to bring lubrication to the tissues. Sour is second best because it is a warming digestive aid. Sweet is third best because it is moisturizing and grounding for vata. Pungent, bitter, and astringent are all tastes that have disadvantages for vata, being dry or cold, so should be minimized.

Recall that pitta is the hot dosha that ups inflammation. To treat pitta, emphasize the cooling tastes—sweet, bitter, and astringent. Limit your use of the hot tastes—sour, salty, and especially pungent. Bitter is best for controlling pitta, as it is very cold. Next is cooling sweet taste. Astringent, also cold, is valuable.

Kapha, as we have seen, is the dosha that increases weight gain and mucus. To treat kapha, focus on the catabolic tastes—pungent, bitter, and astringent. Limit your intake of anabolic sweet, sour, and salty. Pungent is best for kapha because it is dry and hot, while bitter and astringent are both dry.

Most people eat mostly sweet taste because this is the building taste of the macronutrients—proteins, carbohydrates, and fats. Treating vata requires the largest proportion of sweet taste—about 92 percent of the total food consumed. Treating pitta requires about 89 percent sweet, while treating kapha, which already promotes too much sweet, requires a lesser 79 percent.

The other five tastes are provided in the diet by the micronutrients, which are in much smaller dietary proportions.

Most often, the diet that is best for you to achieve balance will be the same as the diet that balances your constitution. However, remember that any dosha can be out of balance at any given time, so you need to treat what you are like *now*.

For example, if you are a thin-framed, always-cold person with dry skin, you have a vata constitution (cold, dry, and light) and should eat as your lifetime program a compensating warm, moist, grounding diet aimed at balancing vata. However, if this week you happen to be retaining water, feel sluggish, and have a chest full of mucus, you are experiencing a temporary kapha imbalance (cold, wet, and heavy) and should eat a compensating warm, dry, light diet until your body is again balanced and healthy.

Food Qualities

The foods you eat will act in your body based on their energy properties, such as temperature, weight, and moisture, as we have discussed. The inherent taste, another way of recognizing biochemical composition, will also be important.

To balance the doshas in your body, identify the dosha that has become overly dominant and is causing problems, For example, if you are feeling sluggish, have put on some weight as fat, and have a consistently stuffy nose, kapha has come to prominence and is overpowering the other two doshas. When you know which dosha needs to be suppressed to bring it back into balance, you can begin to determine which specific foods to emphasize in your daily routine.

Foods for Balancing Kapha

Foods that bring overactive kapha into balance are those with warm, dry, and light qualities. Highlight these in your diet. Avoid foods with opposite energies that would make kapha worse—those that are cold, oily, and heavy. Pungent, bitter, and astringent tastes are catabolic and reduce tissue, which is a good thing, as kapha tends to promote too much tissue growth.

Generally, you should eat less total food, or at least reduce the total fat and calorie content of your diet, to balance kapha. Include warming spices like garlic, black pepper, and chiles, and focus on spicy herbal teas, including ginger. Skip a meal occasionally, or even fast for a day or two from time to time. Eat the largest meal at midday, when the digestive energy is the highest.

For reducing kapha excess in the body, eat dry and astringent fruits. Try cranberries, pomegranates, apples, and raisins. Raw vegetables are low calorie. Also good are cooked beans made with warming spices. When selecting grains, use dry versions, such as rice cakes, whenever possible.

Stay away from oily foods, including nuts. In addition, avoid sweet fruits. Milk products are cold and heavy, so they are not good if you are working on reducing kapha.

Foods for Balancing Pitta

Foods that bring overactive pitta into balance are those with cool, dry, and heavy qualities. Highlight these in your diet. Avoid foods with opposite energies that would make kapha worse—those that are hot, wet, and light. Sweet, bitter, and astringent tastes are cooling and reduce inflammation, a necessity for controlling pitta, as pitta tends to promote too much inflammation.

Generally, you should eat mild foods served raw or cool to balance pitta. Include no warming spices, and keep the oil content low. Focus on cooling herbal teas, including spearmint. Eat when you are calm, and consume three meals at day at regular times.

For reducing kapha excess in the body, try sweet fruits like pears. Sweet and bitter vegetables, such as raw salad greens, also cool down excess pitta. Beans are generally good. Sweet tastes control pitta, so include natural sweeteners like raw sugar and maple syrup in moderation. Also good are mild cheeses such as cottage cheese and sweet, cooling drinks such as apple juice.

Stay away from pungent foods, the main taste category that aggravates pitta. These foods include onion, garlic, and chili peppers. Sour foods and fermented milk products are also out, so nix the yogurt. In addition, avoid oils and nuts.

Foods for Balancing Vata

Foods that bring overactive vata into balance are those with warm, moist, and heavy qualities. Highlight these in your diet. Avoid foods with opposite energies that would make vata worse—those that are cold, dry, and light. Sweet, sour, and salty tastes are anabolic and build tissue—a good thing, as vata tends to cause tissue wasting.

Generally, you should eat more total food—or at least up the oil and calorie contents, if you can comfortably digest this type of diet—to balance vata. Foods to control vata should be filling, nourishing, easy to digest, moistening, and strengthening. Mainly, foods should be cooked to aid digestion. Include mild warming spices like basil, cinnamon, and clove, and focus on herbal teas that promote good digestion, including fennel seed and cardamom seed.

Consume your food warm in small, frequent, regular meals prepared with mild warming spices. Eat in a calm atmosphere, and concentrate while eating.

For reducing vata excess in the body, try sweet fruits. Try cooked apples and apricots. Cook your vegetables. When selecting grains, use cooked mushy preparations. Oatmeal is a great vata-controlling breakfast. It's nourishing, grounding, warm, and easy to digest. Milk products work well to control vata. A glass of warm milk with a little natural sweetener like honey and a mild warming spice like cinnamon is ideal for soothing cold, dry vata problems. Vata dosha is dry, so oil can be used to correct it. Oily foods like nuts are good for bringing vata into balance.

Stay away from foods that produce gas, including beans, melons, and vegetables from the cabbage family. Also avoid dry fruits, dry grains such as rice cakes, and raw vegetables.

Common Herbs for the Doshas

Simple, commonly available herbal medicines and cooking herbs can play a big role in keeping the doshas in balance or in restoring balance if things get out of whack. If you are experiencing symptoms caused by one of the doshas, add selected home herbal medicines to your routine or focus on preparing your diet with the spices that will control the errant dosha and restore balance.

In general, kapha can be balanced with warming, drying herbs like cayenne, garlic, and basil. For pitta, try adding cooling herbs like aloe, spearmint, and dandelion. Excess vata will benefit from warming herbs, including garlic, ginger, and cinnamon. For herbs to use for specific complaints, see Table 2.6.

Table 2.6. Balancing Herbs for Specific Disorders		
	To Balance Kapha	**To Balance Pitta**	**To Balance Vata**
Digestion	Cayenne, black pepper, ginger, cloves	Aloe vera, turmeric, fennel, spearmint	Garlic, ginger, cinnamon, cumin
Elimination (bowels)	Fennel, cardamom	Cascara sagrada, rhubarb root	Psyllium seed, castor oil
Stamina	Garlic, cinnamon, basil	Licorice root, dandelion root	Ginseng, garlic
Mental functions	Sage, basil, scullcap	Sandalwood, hibiscus	Valerian, chamomile

Personalize Your Lifestyle with Ayurveda

Just as we should eat a certain diet according to the dosha we need to balance, we should conduct our life according to the dosha we are seeking to balance. Our schedule, our relationships, our choice of exercise, all can be calculated using Ayurveda.

When Kapha dominates, people are slow and lethargic. They like a lot of sleep and tend toward obesity. To balance kapha:

- *Be active.*
- Participate in stimulating activities.
- Do physical labor.
- Stay warm.
- Sunbathe.
- Get less sleep (sleep fewer hours at night and do not take naps during the day).
- Enjoy a variety of activities.
- Avoid cold and dampness.
- Cultivate physical challenges.
- Pursue mental stimulation.
- Travel as much as possible.
- Avoid being a couch potato.

When pitta dominates, people are hot, intense, aggressive, and demanding. To balance pitta:

- *Be calm.*
- Rest and relax as much as possible.
- Cut down your schedule.
- Cut down on striving.
- Stay cool.
- Take in cool breezes.
- Enjoy flowers, gardens, and gardening.
- Seek contentment.
- Be forgiving.
- Simplify your life.
- Avoid sunlight.
- Enjoy moonlight.

When vata dominates, people are spaced-out, flighty, erratic, anxious, and insomniac. To balance vata:

- *Be moderate.*
- Get adequate sleep.
- Do not stay up late.
- Follow a disciplined schedule.
- Keep regular hours.
- Seek consistency.
- Take in the sun.
- Practice sexual moderation.
- Avoid physical discomfort.
- Avoid wind and cold.
- Avoid overworking.
- Avoid all types of stress.
- Avoid intense travel.
- Avoid excess stimulation, such as from watching television.

Through Ayurveda, the ultimate self-care system, we can help balance our doshas using careful lifestyle choices.

Personalize Your Love Life with Ayurveda

Your relationship can improve if you understand the doshas. Ayurveda suggests a spouse of a different constitution. This helps create balance in the relationship and prevents your offspring from being too extreme in any one dosha. Two vatas would produce a child who is doubly vata, for example.

This goes for the pH perspective, too. If you are constitutionally quite acid, for example, and you marry someone who is also on the acid side, your children will likely be even more acidic for their lifetimes.

To achieve balance in your love life, there are a number of things you can do. To balance kapha:

- Marry a vata.
- Enjoy an active family life.
- Engage in stimulating conversations.
- Encourage talking.
- Go out and find things that interest you.
- Encourage sexual interest.

To balance pitta:

- Marry a kapha or vata.
- Keep your conversations soothing.
- Avoid confrontation.
- Share relaxing massages.
- Take "cool off" breaks.
- Take time and care with sex.

To balance vata:

- Marry a kapha.
- Develop your relationship slowly and steadily.
- Think less, act more.
- Take care in managing your money.
- Welcome commitment.
- Practice consistent and supportive behavior.
- Be cautious in sexual experimentation.
- Don't overtalk and don't overanalyze.

Personalize Your Exercise Routine with Ayurveda

Your exercise program can go a long way toward balancing your doshas or keeping them in balance. Kapha dosha is slow and heavy, so if it dominates, you will gain weight and feel sluggish. To balance kapha:

- Do hot workouts.
- Exercise in a warm environment.
- Push yourself to get hot and sweat.
- Emphasize vigorous aerobic activities and powerful calisthenics.
- Push your limits.
- Practice discipline to combat laziness.

Pitta is the hot dosha, so it will cause you to overheat easily if it dominates. To balance pitta:

- Do moderate workouts.
- Don't allow yourself to become overheated.
- Dress lightly.
- Work out in cool air.
- Don't be fanatical—take plenty of cool-down breaks.
- Drink plenty of water.
- Vary your routine to avoid boredom.

Vata is the dosha that produces frailty, cold, and fatigue. To balance vata:

- Do mild workouts.
- Stay warm while you exercise.
- Dress warmly, even if it means wearing heavier clothing than those around you.
- Find a good routine and stick with it.
- Increase the intensity of your routine slowly and gradually.
- Don't overdo it; avoid undue fatigue.
- Stick with easy stretching, walking, mild yoga.

Dosha Cycles and pH

According to Ayurveda, each dosha has a time in your life when it is prone to dominate your body energy. Everyone, regardless of his or her individual constitution, is under the exaggerated effects of that dosha during that time of life.

During childhood, kapha dominates. During these years, everyone feels the effects of the cold, wet, heavy energy. It helps build the body you will live in for the rest of your life. Childhood is an alkaline time. You can eat more hot acid foods.

When puberty strikes as a hormone tornado, we heat up and pitta begins to dominate. Pitta continues to rise until it peaks at around age forty, then it begins a long, slow decline. This is the high-acid time of life. It's the time of midlife stress. Hot, wet, light pitta pushes all of us. Consume cooling alkaline foods during this time.

By about age sixty, vata catches up with pitta and begins to dominate. Regardless of our individual constitution, we all eventually get colder, lighter, and drier. You can go back to enjoying a higher proportion of warming acidic foods.

Ayurveda is probably the oldest continuously practiced healing system on the planet. Over many generations, people have had a very long and consistent opportunity to experiment with their health programs, make adjustments, and experience the results. Centuries of experimentation and a huge, growing knowledge base have created a remarkably effective system of health assessment and treatment. Ayurveda is particularly good at predicting the likely consequences of any lifestyle, food, or behavior. You can know, with considerable certainty, what will happen to your health next week, next year, and in the next decade when you eat a certain food today. The great thing about Ayurveda is that all the relevant body chemistry considerations are wrapped up in the holistic overview of the body's energies. You don't need to perform a bunch of complicated tests or have a technical understanding of chemistry. The signs from your own body give you an integrated method of putting together a huge range of information in a cohesive way.

Ayurveda also provides a systematic way to get immediate feedback from your body. When you calculate the balance of the doshas and set about creating a change, you can figure out pretty quickly whether you are getting the results you expect by checking your experience against the dosha scheme. If you are proceeding toward balance, you are on the right track and can expect to get good results. If things are not going the way you planned, you can evaluate the results you are experiencing and tweak your strategy to adjust the dosha energies.

Body Balance will bring you back to wellness and keep you well. Ayurveda, with its extensive scheme of body typing, can be an integral part of that journey.

3

The Flowing Tao: Balance in East Asian Traditional Medicine

As we embark on the journey to lifelong good health and body balance, it helps to get some different perspectives. Looking at a situation through a different lens can sometimes illuminate a critical aspect of health that you have been missing.

Chinese medicine is one of the two oldest established paradigms of herbal medicine still being practiced. It is a truly holistic system that has diagnosed and treated disease for at least 3,000 years. More importantly, it has kept hundreds of generations of people well and healthy, preventing untold suffering.

Centuries of formulation of theories, and testing of these theories in practice, have resulted in the system we today recognize as Traditional Chinese Medicine (TCM). Based on the principles of balance and harmony, this highly sophisticated and complex discipline works to heal and regenerate the body's organs and systems. TCM considers humans to be mini-ecosystems—organic wholes—that share common traits with the environment in which they live, so that changes in the natural environment may directly or indirectly affect them. For example, a change of seasons or the cycling from day to night may change the body's condition. In order to attain and maintain health, TCM considers not only what goes into the patient, but what goes on around the patient.

In TCM, the vital energy known as *qi* (pronounced CHEE) is the basis of all life. It is the universal life energy in every living creature. This energy circulates throughout the body to every cell and organ. In the body, qi is accumulated, distributed, and eventually eliminated. All health depends on the proper balance of qi.

TCM is based on a broad categorization of energy into two opposing yet complementary categories: yin (cooling) and yang (warming) energies. All TCM theories and practices start with these basic concepts of yin and yang. In TCM, which is similar to Ayurveda, herbs, foods, and other natural medicines are categorized by their temperature, taste, and action on the body, such as moving the blood, dispelling dampness or heat, breaking up stagnation, or building stamina. TCM traditionally also includes remedies made from animals, such as deer antler, and mineral medicines, such as gypsum, as healing substances. TCM considers each remedy's energetic makeup along with that of the patient, so that the energetics can be precisely matched, resulting in a more holistic approach to healing.

In China, TCM was becoming overshadowed by Western scientific medicine by the nineteenth and early twentieth centuries. However, the Communist revolution in the mid-twentieth century revived TCM as "a national treasure," in the words of Mao. Then, under the influence of materialistic communism, TCM underwent a transition from its more obvious earlier spiritual, mystical, Taoist influences to a more strictly physical approach. In this Communist form, it has enjoyed increasing favor throughout many Western countries. Many Western practitioners today, though, feel a need to reinvestigate the universal spiritual orientation of original TCM.

In America, there has been widespread acceptance of acupuncture in recent years. It has been licensed in the majority of the states. Fortunately, this has opened the door for people's interest in other TCM techniques, including herbalism.

Renowned herbalist and acupuncturist Michael Tierra says, "After decades of practice and study of Western, Native American, and Ayurvedic systems of medicine, I feel that with its integrated theoretical, diagnostic, and medicinal classification system and over 3,000 years of accumulated experience, Traditional Chinese Medicine is indeed the most effective system of healing and a truly worthy alternative to Western scientific allopathy."

Chinese Energetics

Ancient Chinese physicians had only their own insight and the acuity of their senses to grasp an impression about the nature of a patient's health and to reach a conclusion about which protocol to apply. So, the manner in which they detailed health imbalances and the nomenclature they created to catalog the assorted patterns of disharmony were obviously different from contemporary conventions. They did not acknowledge microbial diseases because they did not have the modern tools to identify microbes and to associate them with symptom complexes. This does not mean, however, that they lacked effective means to deal with microbial infections. Just because they did not explicitly state that a cold is caused by a virus does not mean that they could not effectively prevent or treat the symptoms of a cold. The energetic classifications they used to systematize acute disharmonies permitted them to select fitting herbal protocols, diets, and acupuncture treatments for a particular imbalance with great utility.

The TCM system of healthcare begins with a differentiation of the individual's energetic situation, starting with the most basic divisions, and extends the process of differentiation to a great degree of specificity. Chinese physicians have found the Five Elements of TCM philosophy alone to be insufficient to characterize the variety and intricacy of disharmonies that can manifest in any given person. As a result, over the last two millennia they have developed more detailed theories and taxonomy of categories of illness, capable of encompassing the reality of disease individualization seen in clinical practice.

Qi

TCM is based on the principle of unconditional energy of all phenomena. Called *qi*, or *chi*, it is ephemeral, active, constantly changing, and warm. Qi is the basis of all organic life, and of all inorganic substances as well. Qi is vital energy. When you are young and energetic, you have abundant qi, but as your qi declines with age, you become subject to degenerative diseases and lowered vitality. This concept of qi is the basis for the success of TCM in the area of health maintenance and longevity.

In the Chinese view, the primary principle of health is recognizing and promoting the flow of qi and eliminating its blockage. All TCM techniques, including herbs, diet, and acupuncture, are aimed at this result.

Yin and Yang

The *I Ching*, or *Book of Changes*, ascribed to Lao Tzu (circa 1250 B.C.), contains the first known mention of the philosophy of yin and yang. Energies that characterize the complementary yet opposing materialization of all phenomena, yin and yang are the most basic divisions of energy in the universe. That which is above corresponds to something below; heat is complemented by cold, night is pursued by day. In all of manifest creation, qi is divided and apparent in duality. All matter and energy in the universe can be represented on the spectrum of yin merging into yang.

Translated, *yin* comes from the "shady side of the mountain" and *yang* from the "sunny side of the mountain."

Health is yin and yang in balance.

Yin and Yang Qualities

Yin and yang are the polar opposites of a continuum of energy. For each energy characteristic, yin has a quality and yang has the opposite quality. For example, yin is quiet, while yang is active. The ideal balance in the body is in the middle. We don't want to be too calm or too active. A person in whom yin dominates will have a tendency to be quiet and calm, while a person in whom yang dominates will tend toward being active.

The yin, quiet person should be given treatments to move him or her more toward yang. A good herbal treatment would be the herb ginseng, for example. The yang person should be treated with remedies to move the energy toward yin. In this case, black sesame seed would be a good example.

For additional yin and yang qualities, see Table 3.1.

Yin and Yang Constitution

The polarity of yin and yang are reflected even in the basic makeup of a person's body. From birth, these energies have the tendency to be established in the body in a proportionate balance; people tip one way or the other. People with a yin constitution will have a body that is cold and wet. They will have soft, delicate, flaccid features; a soft voice; and a

Table 3.1. Yin and Yang Qualities	
Yin	**Yang**
Conserves	Radiates
Quiet	Active
Concentrated	Expanded
Descending	Ascending
Internal	External
Feminine	Masculine
Receptive	Aggressive
Timid	Bold
Night	Day
Cold	Hot
Wet	Dry
Heavy	Light
Dark	Bright

pale complexion. They will likely suffer from fatigue and low blood pressure. Their yang counterparts will have a body that is hot and dry. They will have coarse features, firm tissues, a loud voice, and a flushed complexion. They will likely be hyperactive and suffer from high blood pressure.

Yin and Yang in TCM Diagnosis

We can even use the yin and yang energies to aid in diagnosis of disease. Yin diseases (for which yang remedies are used) occur deep in the body, are accompanied by feelings of cold, involve fatigue and under-nourishment, and tend to be chronic in nature. Yang diseases (for which yin remedies are used) have symptoms that appear on the surface of the body, are hot, involve overactivity and accumulation of tissue or wastes, and tend to be acute in nature.

The Three Humors

The yin-yang energy spectrum can be further subdivided into energies dubbed qi, blood, and moisture. In the body, all functions are the result of interactions of qi, blood, and moisture. We need all these functions in order to have a functional body. The three humors, as these energies are called, are interdependent, and they are all generated from our environment in a harmonious balance. This holistic system of interactive humors allows each humor to be involved in the regulation of the other two.

Qi is associated with yang, while blood is associated with yin. In TCM, qi is deemed "the commander of blood," and blood is "the mother of qi," so there is an interdependent connection between them, mirroring the relationship of yin with yang. Men are more likely to have qi disorders, whereas women will have more blood problems.

Qi is the essential energy of the being, of life. It is an immaterial force.

We take in qi through the air we breathe and the food we eat. It is the basic forming and organizing principle in life, so it regulates the fundamental shape of the body we live in and it supplies the energy to enliven the body and allow it to be active. Thus it is responsible for the total vitality we are granted to live our life and is even ultimately responsible for the lifespan. When the qi is gone, life is over.

When qi begins to wane, the symptoms are fatigue and weakness, with shortness of breath. Timid behavior, a soft voice, and pale skin are all signs of loss of qi. Qi deficiency often causes digestive disturbance characterized by gas.

TCM has identified several herbs as "qi tonics," which help to replenish declining qi. They include ginseng, astragalus, and cardamom.

While qi is an energy that cannot be seen, blood is actually a material substance. The blood humor is similar in concept to the Western idea of blood. It nurtures, moistens, and lubricates the tissues. Its job is to generate tissue and to distribute and store nutrients. Folks with blood deficiency experience pale skin, scanty menstruation, anemia, dizziness, and insomnia. Blood-building herbs are dong quai and rehmannia.

Moisture, sometimes translated as "essence," or *jing*, corresponds to an additional refinement from a grosser material. *Jing* comprises all the fluids in our body except the blood. It includes the intracellular fluids and the extracellular fluids, including the lymph. It is a material substance, but it is not contained in any particular form as it seeps throughout the body, so it is called amorphous. The *jing* fluids are formed from the foods and beverages we consume. Moisture is considered to have two basic actions in the body. First, it moistens tissues such as the skin and mucus membranes. Second, it seeps into the blood and is carried to all the parts of the body, moistening all the tissues.

People with a lack of adequate moisture humor develop dry membranes, including skin and eyes, and constipation. Apricot seed is a classic moisturizing herb.

For a comparison of the characteristics and deficiency symptoms of the three humors, see Table 3.2.

The Five Elements

The Chinese Five Elements symbolize interactive energies that are primary to the natural cycles of existence. Originally, they were probably a further division of yin-yang relationships. Essentially that is a good way to conceive of them. They are metaphorical concepts that allow us to conceptualize the infinite possible ways that matter and energy can interact in the universe. The five elements in TCM are fire, earth, metal, water, and wood.

Fire element bears the power of warmth and expansion. It is hot, causes upward movement in the body, is light, and is a source of energy for metabolism. Foods and herbs rich in fire element give the body heat, help to generate healthy blood, and promote circulation.

Earth element is associated with nourishment. In the body, earth element is responsible for digestion, transformation, and transportation of food. Substances with sweet taste, such as whole grains, most vegetables, meat, licorice, and honey, contain earth element.

Metal element signifies the power of solidity and the energy of receiving and discharging. In the body, it receives and controls vital energy

Table 3.2. The Three Humors		
	Qi	**Blood**	**Moisture**
Characteristics	Essential energy Breath/air Body shape Body activity Forming/organizing Immaterial force Total vitality/lifespan	Tissue generation Nutrient distribution Nutrient storage	Tissue lubrication Skin moistening Internal environment Fluid generation Fluid distribution Amorphous substance
Symptoms of deficiency	Fatigue Weakness Shortness of breath Timidity Soft voice Paleness Dizziness Tinnitus Palpitations Perspiration Gas Weak digestion Low appetite White, moist tongue coating	Paleness Scanty menstruation Anemia Pale skin and lips Dizziness Insomnia Numbness	Dryness Constipation
Herbs to nourish	Ginseng Astragalus Codonopsis Dioscorea Pinellia Citrus peel Cardamom	Rehmannia Dong quai Lycii berry	Apricot seed

and eliminates waste, so it is associated with the lungs and the large intestine. Foods and herbs with a pungent, spicy taste increase metal element and enhance the functions of respiration and elimination through the bowels.

Water element is characterized by fluidity. It is associated with love and all the sense processes. It regulates water balance, so it is connected with the kidneys and bladder. It stores jing. Water element nourishes the brain and bone marrow. Substances with a salty taste, such as kelp, contain water element.

Wood element represents growth and flexibility. It stores blood and regulates the smooth flow of qi. Medicines with a sour taste are rich in wood element.

Temperature

TCM also organizes the clinical actions of herbs and foods by temperature, which is probably the most basic and significant type of energy in an herb or food. The TCM classification of temperature is subjective and based on qualities in the patient's reaction to the substance. TCM has five major temperature classifications: cold, cool, neutral, warm, and hot. For example, watermelon is cold, salad vegetables are cool, rice is neutral, fresh ginger is warm, and dried ginger is hot.

This fivefold scheme gives us a better grasp of food and herb temperature effects than the two designations in Ayurveda, so people often find it a bit easier to apply.

Hot characteristics in foods and herbs increase metabolic rate and open circulation throughout the body. They raise body temperature, speed up chemical reactions, and burn more nutrients. The more nutrients we burn, the more acids we produce that have to be chemically neutralized in the body. Hot substances are inflammatory over time. Heat burns up tissues and is considered catabolic.

Cold foods slow down metabolic rate and suppress circulation. They lower body temperature and slow metabolic reactions. Because cold suppresses metabolism, fewer nutrients are burned and therefore less acid is liberated, resulting in the body having less acid stress to neutralize. But if the body is too cold, it can't burn nutrients to run essential functions.

Watermelon will cool you down, as anyone who has gone to a summer picnic can attest.

Taste

Taste represents a sensory method of ascertaining the biochemical action of a given herb or food—in other words, the remedy's "energy."

TCM has five tastes: pungent, salty, sour, bitter, and sweet. (See Table 3.3.) Each taste represents the content of various chemical constituents and offers distinct energy effects.

Pungent taste is the bite you get from onions and chiles. Pungent-tasting herbs usually contain volatile oils. Their energy is hot. Pungency increases digestion, circulation, perspiration, and saliva. Pungent taste is used in TCM to promote sweating in the treatment of skin diseases. Cinnamon and ginger are pungent herbs.

Salty stabilizes fluid balance in the body by balancing the amount of water retention in the tissues. Salty taste is cold. It softens and frees masses, including swollen lymph nodes and various lumps. Kelp is a salty food.

Sour stimulates digestion and bile secretion, as well as drying mucus. Sour taste is cooling in TCM. Foods with a sour taste produce their action through organic acids. Acidic foods tend to be high in vitamin content. Rose hips are sour therapy, contain vitamin C, and are used for the respiratory tract. Sour foods can increase acid load. The TCM definition of sour includes the category that Ayurveda calls astringent. Astringency is usually caused by tannins in the food. Citrus peels are used to promote digestion and stimulate appetite. Schisandra berry is a classic TCM tonic herb that is primarily sour.

Bitter is a cold, drying taste. It is the ultimate detoxifying taste, and it promotes the secretion of digestive juices from the upper gastrointestinal tract, aiding digestion. TCM uses bitter taste to fight infection and inflammation. Gentian root and rhubarb root are bitter. Bitter-tasting substances tend to be alkaline.

Sweet taste is the builder. Sweet-tasting plants' active compounds are often carbohydrates or amino acids. This cooling taste is responsible for nourishing and building tissue. Sweet herbs are tonics that increase stamina. Ginseng and astragalus are sweet herbs.

The Four Diagnoses

According to TCM, proper diagnosis is supreme. Without accurate diagnosis, all therapy is trial and error. TCM diagnosis is subtle and complex. Primarily, it is based on the Four Diagnoses: observation, palpation, interrogation, and listening.

Observation takes in such issues as eyes, complexion, posture, and

Table 3.3. The Five Tastes				
Taste	Energy (Temperature)	Organs (Elements) Affected	Properties	Comments
Pungent	Hot	Lung and large intestine	Increases digestion, circulation, perspiration, and saliva	For surface conditions
Salty	Cold	Kidney, adrenal glands, and bladder	Stabilizes fluid balance and softens lymph nodes, constipation, lumps, tight muscles, and cysts	
Sour	Cold, dry	Liver and gallbladder	Dries mucus, tightens tissue (astringent), and stimulates digestion and bile	Ayurveda further divides this into bitter and astringent
Bitter	Cold, dry	Heart and small intestine	Dries, detoxifies, reduces inflammation, and promotes bile, digestion, and bowel movement	
Sweet	Cold	Spleen and stomach	Builds, harmonizes, tonifies, and nourishes	

body movement. The practitioner also looks for clues to underlying energy imbalances in the hair, body shape and configuration, and emotional expressiveness. In addition, the practitioner inspects the tongue for thickness, color, coating, and the appearance and consistency of the surrounding tissue.

Palpation focuses primarily on the pulse and all the energy indications TCM draws from this complicated study. TCM pulse evaluation expands on conventional medical technique. In addition to the pulse rate, the tactile features in three positions over the left and right radial pulse are noted. Both tongue and pulse qualities are extremely sensitive indicators of ill health, and practiced investigators are usually able to correlate abnormal deviations with symptoms well before an imbalance results in clinically abnormal blood chemistry or X rays. Gross deviations from normal in pulse and tongue characteristics usually indicate severe imbalances verifiable by medical evaluation.

To a lesser extent, the TCM practitioner may also palpate body cavities and extremities.

Interrogation is asking systematic questions of the patient. The TCM practitioner begins by evaluating the patient's list of complaints, all the while taking in the patient's general appearance and demeanor. Every nuance is assessed based on principles of yin and yang.

The practitioner asks ten basic questions covering symptoms that are not otherwise obvious. The answers help the practitioner to form an impression. The ten questions concern the following areas:

1. Chills, fever, and sensitivity to heat and cold
2. Perspiration—night sweats, easy perspiring on mild exertion, etc.
3. Pain anywhere in the body
4. Elimination (urination and defecation)—frequency, color, etc.
5. Appetite and food cravings
6. Mental health—depression, anxiety, etc.
7. Hearing—acuity, tinnitus, etc.
8. Thirst
9. Personal and family health history, and any personal insights from the patient
10. Menstrual and reproductive history

The aim of asking the questions is to ascertain patterns underlying the symptoms to determine the cause of the disharmony. TCM considers no condition untreatable. All disharmonies are based in energy imbalances, and the balance of energy always has a chance of being improved.

The Eight Principles of Diagnosis

The Eight Principles of Diagnosis combine to form the most basic diagnostic tool in TCM and are almost always adequate for ascertaining a complete approach to treatment.

This technique is the key to beginning treatment according to pattern identification. This exemplifies the oft-quoted maxim "one disease, many formulas; one formula, many diseases." A specific patient can be treated properly only according to a holistic differential diagnosis. In addition, a single herbal formula may be used for treating several diseases with different Western names, but with similar energy disruptions.

The Eight Principles offer a comparatively straightforward approach to interpreting the overall yin-yang balance of the body. Further refinement of the diagnosis brings us to the specificity needed for the individual case.

The Eight Principles consist of three pairs of energy indications (exterior-interior, cold-hot, and deficiency-excess) and an overall synopsis of the body energy as reflected in the first two (yin-yang). (See Table 3.4.)

Assigning the Treatment

The therapeutic foundation of TCM is to reduce or tonify or to regulate yin and yang. Every disorder is fundamentally an imbalance of one or both of these factors.

A diet or herb's effect on the body is eventually determined by the dose and the unique condition of the patient using it.

Taste, of course, is one way of deciding which herbs have the needed actions.

Bitter remedies, such as gentian, can be used in small doses before meals as digestive preparations, stimulating secretion of digestive juices and provoking both appetite and efficient digestion. Bitter taste is cold, so it is used to "clear heat"—that is, reduce inflammation, which is associated with acidity in Western terms.

Table 3.4. The Eight Principles of Diagnosis		
Principle	**Symptoms**	**Treatment**
Yin	Paleness, fatigue, shortness of breath, weak voice, loose stool, clear urine	Warm, tonify
Yang	Flushing, restlessnes, loud voice, rapid breathing, dark urine, constipation	Cool, sedate
Internal	No visible symptoms	Variable (other factors)
External	Fever, chills, aversion to wind and cold	Expel, perspire
Cold	Aversion to cold, cold extremities, paleness, lack of thirst, clear urine, loose stool	Warm, dispel cold
Hot	Aversion to heat, hot extremities, thirst, preference for cold drinks, nervousness, dark urine, constipation	Cool, sedate
Empty	Fatigue, shortness of breath, low resistance, poor appetite, weight loss	Tonify
Full	Overactivity, restlessness, loud voice, harsh breathing, abdominal distention, dark urine, constipation	Scatter, expel, purge

Salty foods, such as seaweeds, bring out the yang flavor of food and provoke a yang effect in the body. They help retain fluids, moisten tissue, and support the kidneys.

Sour taste is found in foods containing organic acids. Sour taste enhances digestion, especially of proteins. It also enhances liver function.

Sweet taste is nourishing, so it is used to tonify. The waste by-products of this building process are acid, though, so we need to be conscious of keeping the body pH-balanced when we are in a rebuilding, or healing, phase.

Spicy taste stimulates, warms, and dries dampness. It is used in conditions of excess dampness (mucus) in the lungs, which are associated with the metal element.

The Eight Methods of Herbal Treatment

TCM seeks to balance the body by selecting the way in which a medicine will act. Chinese physicians have identified eight procedures that produce physiological changes in the body and result in adjustments in the body's energetics. These eight methods are sweating, stomach cleansing, purgation, harmonizing, warming and cooling, removing (detoxifying), tonification, and reducing. (See Table 3.5.) When a TCM practitioner puts together a treatment program, he or she decides which method or combination of methods is appropriate to the case and selects foods and herbs that will have that action.

Sweating

Use sweating therapy for external conditions—principally, cold and fever. While TCM uses exterior releasing as a strategy to treat skin disease, it is usually not a practical option with Americans, as it tends to cause the skin symptoms to temporarily worsen before improving and Americans have no way of discerning that they are not, in fact, actually getting permanently worse.

Stomach Cleansing

Stomach cleansing is one therapy that will likely be slow in catching on in the West. In TCM, vomiting therapy is used mainly as an emergency measure for poisoning, much as it is in the United States. TCM often uses a strong licorice tea to induce vomiting. In the West, we usually use syrup of ipecac.

Purgation

Purgation is used to eliminate an excess of waste material through the large intestine. Laxative remedies are used in patterns of excess charac-

Table 3.5. The Eight Methods of Herbal Treatment				
Method	**Indications**	**Applications**	**Comments**	**Contra-indications**
Sweating	External conditions (skin diseases and other energy blocks close to body surface)	Colds and fever	"External" refers to the epithelial tissue, even though the condition may be within the body. If using sweating and purging (for chills, fever, headache, and stiffness with constipation), first sweat, then purge	Serious body-fluid loss
Stomach cleansing	Food poisoning, mucus accumulation	Lung congestion, abdominal pain	Rarely used to reduce accumulated mucus. Use with slippery herbs, e.g., licorice	Substances that would cause damage if regurgitated
Purgation	Excess conditions, constipation, pelvic pain, intestinal parasites	Elimination of toxins through colon, intestinal parasites	Two types: (1) using bitter and cool herbs and foods (e.g., rhubarb root), and (2) using warm herbs and foods (e.g., daphne flower)	Fluid loss, frailty, menstruation, pregnancy, postpartum, external conditions

Table 3.5. The Eight Methods of Herbal Treatment (Continued)				
Method	Indications	Applications	Comments	Contra-indications
Harmonizing	Yang diseases of liver, gall-bladder, and stomach	General imbalance, fever, chest pain, nausea, hot diseases (e.g., malaria), thirst, PMS with edema and mood swings	Most common TCM herbal method	Clearly defined condition
Warming	Cold conditions	Coldness, vomiting, weakness, abdominal pain, weak pulse, weak digestion, loose stools, clear urine, cold extremities, poor appetite, abdominal distension, stomach pains	Strengthens yang qi	Excess heat, internal heat with external chills, spitting up blood, blood in stools, diarrhea with fever
Removing	Blood toxicity	Toxicity, fever, pathogens	Equivalent to "alternatives" (blood cleansers)	Frailty, cold extremities, anxiety
Tonification	Undernourishment	Fatigue, shallow breathing, low fever	Typically uses ginseng and similar herbs	Excess conditions, qi stagnation
Reducing	Blocked qi	Abdominal swelling, obesity, tumors, ulcers	Detoxifying (removes undesirable materials)	Low-grade fever, thirst, diarrhea, weak digestion, blood loss, amenorrhea

terized by stomach and intestinal pains, constipation, dry stools, and stagnant blood in the lower abdomen. Purgatives are contraindicated, from the TCM point of view, in external conditions because they draw the corrupt energy back inward. TCM prefers to release it. However, Americans usually do not tolerate the side effects in the exterior tissues (skin rash).

Harmonizing

Harmonizing is the most frequently indicated herbal treatment in TCM. It is used primarily for disorders of the liver, gallbladder, and stomach energy systems. In mixed conditions, where no clear symptom pattern is apparent, it is the treatment of choice—when some symptoms are internal and some are external, for instance. Another example is persistent cold and fever involving mixed external and internal, hot and cold, and excess and deficiency symptoms.

Warming and Cooling

Warming is a method used to enhance and fortify yang qi. It is often indicated in hypoglycemia, hypothyroidism, and hypoadrenalism. The inverse method, cooling, is used in inflammation and fevers.

Removing (Detoxifying)

Removing therapy uses detoxifying, "blood purifying" herbs and foods. (These are sometimes called "alternatives.") This treatment method lowers fever and destroys pathogens, while leaving valuable body fluids intact. Since removing therapy removes pathogens that cause infection and reduces fever, it is sometimes called "clearing heat." TCM does not use removing therapy if a person has delicate health, cold extremities, diarrhea, anxiety, or extreme physical depletion.

Tonification

Tonification is for deficient, weak patients who need energy and nutrient supplementation. Signs of the need for tonification are fatigue, shallow breathing, pale skin, dizziness, thirst, night sweats, insomnia, chills, lower backache, and impotence. Generally, ginseng and similar herbs are used.

Reducing

Reducing removes qi, blood, or phlegm stagnation. Its aim is similar to that of purgation therapy, but it dissolves accumulations, including cysts, tumors, abnormal swellings, body and blood fat, and blood clots. Reducing treatment is slower than purgation. Often, the therapy is carried out over months.

Using the Eight Methods Clinically

When TCM practitioners apply the eight treatment methods, they must consider which method to do first and what sequence of methods is appropriate for the given patient. These nuances often spell the difference between comfortable success in therapy and less than ideal results.

Any method that eliminates wastes or fluids from the body can be stressful, so the patient must be robust enough to handle the effect of the eliminating therapy. Generally, it's important to tonify any weakness the patient might have before doing purging and stomach cleansing.

TCM says to treat the branch before the root—in other words, don't take on too big a project. This means treating external diseases like skin eruptions and flu before getting down to the deep imbalances in the core of the body. Complicated conditions might require different, potentially conflicting protocols over time. It's wise to proceed cautiously at first, until it becomes a bit more obvious how the treatment is going to work.

If you are undertaking a very long project, which could be called "constitutional treatment," you might need to use TCM methods for years before finally bringing the body into balance. If an acute crisis, like the flu, develops in the meantime, stop the constitutional treatment and handle the acute situation. Once the temporary situation has improved, go back to treating the root issues.

Patients do not need to feel miserable while they are getting better. If side effects occur from a treatment, dosages can always be reduced and treatments taken a little slower. Since body energies change as the days go by, it's important to reevaluate at appropriate intervals. For an acute disease, like the flu, this can be done every couple of days. For constitutional treatments, monthly reevaluations are more typical.

TCM frequently starts any treatment program with a short course of purgation to get the digestive tract cleared out before other medicine goes in. Tonification medicines are taken before meals to enhance absorption, while eliminating remedies are taken after meals to help with detoxification. Also, it's important to coordinate the entire health program. It wouldn't make any sense to use herbs that are countered by the food in the regular diet.

Using the Eight Methods in Combination

There are just a few rules for using the eight methods in combination. If you're miserable with the flu, with fever, chills, headache, and constipation, you have a virus in you. From the TCM point of view, a virus is an undesirable energy that needs to get out. So, we use methods that get undesirable energy out: sweating and purgation. In this case, to avoid getting further depleted, you should sweat before purging.

While you have that nasty flu, if you have fever with chills, you might want to use cooling herbs to reduce the fever. Cooling herbs generally are depleting and make you fatigued, however. So, paradoxically, you might sometimes want to use warming herbs afterward to offset the enfeebling result of the cooling herbs.

Another conundrum that can occur is that you can be weak and simultaneously have a congestion of energy in your body—benign cysts or a blood clot, say. The proper therapy for congested energy is purgation, but purgation is weakening to the general vitality. So, you should split the difference: Do a balanced combination of nourishing therapy for the weakness and moderate purgation for the congestion.

TCM and Body Balance

The TCM concepts of yin and yang are considerably more complex than simple acid-alkaline distinctions. However, they provide a starting point.

Acid is essentially yang, while alkaline is essentially yin. Yang is hot. Yin is cool.

We can start to apply TCM ideas by looking at cooling versus warming foods. Cooling foods are usually alkalinizing and slow down metabolism, reducing the acid load. They reduce inflammation. Foods that are cooling in the TCM system include fruits such as apple, banana, pear, melon, tomato, and citrus; vegetables such as cucumber (very cooling), celery, asparagus, spinach, mild squashes, cabbage, cauliflower, bok choy, lettuce, and dandelion greens; beans such as soy and mung; grains such as millet, wheat, amaranth, and barley; and herbs such as cilantro, red clover, nettle, and mints.

As we age and wear and tear takes its toll on our bodies, we begin to dry out. This loss of juice causes pain, stiffness, constipation, and dry skin. In TCM, this is explained as loss of yin. To stay young and healthy, we should include foods that build yin (the watery, lubricating energy). These are especially effective cooked as a warm soup. Good examples are barley, wheat, rice, quinoa, tofu, black beans, beets, and banana.

TCM is one of the most widely practiced and most respected natural healthcare paradigms in the world. It is used by more people than any other holistic healing system. The main focus of TCM is finding balance and harmony in the body and mind, and sustaining that balance.

Over the centuries, TCM has worked out a very systematic approach to understanding health and balance. It has evolved a specific and detailed method of regaining balance and an explicit strategy for doing so. In TCM, knowing if you're on the right track or not is pretty straightforward. If you follow the principles, it really works.

One of the great things about TCM is that every aspect of your lifestyle is taken into consideration and integrated into the evaluation and treatment. What you eat, which herbs you take, your job, your relationships, all need to be considered and balanced to find a cure. Since you are a mini-ecosystem that interacts with the environmental ecosystem, nothing can be left out of the equation.

Even though TCM is a huge system and is practiced at a very high level by professionals, the basic principles are pretty clear-cut. You can develop a basic understanding of how to apply these techniques and see the results in your life in short order. In this book, we are looking at the challenge of balancing body chemistry through many different lenses. TCM, one of the most well developed and broad in scope, can be a foundational part of your journey toward lifelong health.

4

Macrobiotics: Refining the Balance

Chinese medicine is a huge science that no one could master in a life-time. Truly a system of complete holistic healthcare, it encompasses literally every aspect of human life. TCM assumes that we should be striving for balance in all things and that prevention of disease is far superior to rushing around to treat symptoms after they appear. That's where macrobiotics fits in.

This modern Asian health method focuses on the everyday things we can do to stay healthy. It presents an easy-to-understand theory of yin and yang that we all can apply in our daily lives. The attention of macrobiotics is mainly on food, so it has a well-developed dietary philosophy and eating plan. Macrobiotic teachers have delved into the modern area of pH and correlated these modern chemical concepts with ancient Asian energetics in an interesting way. Let's see how we can expand the concepts we have developed so far, as we continue on our journey toward body balance.

Macrobiotic Basics

Macrobiotics is a modern-day adaptation, a simplification, of the fundamental concepts of Traditional Chinese Medicine. Macrobiotics, as it is practiced today, is based on the teachings and vision of George Ohsawa (1893 to 1966), a Japanese health practitioner. The name of the system comes from the Greek *macro*, meaning "great," and *bios*, meaning "life."

Practitioners describe it as a tool that teaches how to live within the natural order of life and the constantly changing natural world in which we find ourselves. Macrobiotic principles (such as an understanding of yin and yang) can be applied to all areas of life.

The macrobiotic approach to diet focuses on whole grains and fresh vegetables and avoids meat (this is where it departs somewhat from typical TCM), milk products, and processed foods. The body is always adapting to changes in the environment and is always aging, which macrobiotics takes into account. The goal of macrobiotics is to continually balance the effects of influences on the body, primarily through diet, and to regulate these changes in a controlled and peaceful manner.

A basic precept of macrobiotic thinking is that all things are composed of yin and yang energies, but with either yin or yang in excess. According to macrobiotic proponents, most of the standard American foods have very strong yin (white sugar) or yang (red meat) characters, and *also tend to be acid-forming*. Macrobiotic practice, though, emphasizes the two food groups that have the least extreme yin and yang qualities (grains and vegetables), so it is easier for the adherent to achieve a more balanced condition. Balancing a very yang burger with a very yin bowl of ice cream would not be solid macrobiotic practice. Macrobiotics practitioners say that the resulting sense of control is one of the most important benefits of macrobiotic practice. You can actually feel the effects of putting the theory into practice.

Macrobiotic Classification of Foods

As in all Asian healing, balance is the key in macrobiotics. Use Table 4.1 to begin selecting foods that will keep you in solid balance from day to day. Concentrate mainly on foods in the neutral column, such as carrots, oats, and kidney beans, as they are neither too yin nor too yang. If your metabolism leans toward the yin side, you may be a little more generous with yang-producing foods, such as eggs. Remember, most folks are too acid and yang foods tend to be acidifying, so a little of these yang foods goes a long way. In general, macrobiotics does not favor using red meat.

If you are too far to the yang side, you may allow yourself more yin-producing foods. But take a look at the list. Many of the yin-producing foods, such as alcoholic beverages and ice cream, are nutrient empty.

Table 4.1. Yin, Yang, and Neutral Foods		
Yin Foods	**Neutral Foods**	**Yang Foods**
Alcoholic beverages	Barley	Cabbage
Bananas	Burdock	Eggs
Butter	Carrots	Fowl
Celery	Corn	Mustard greens
Citrus fruits	Daikon	Red meats
Fruit juices (in general)	Garlic	Shellfish
Ice cream	Kidney beans	
Lettuce	Most vegetables, especially	
Milk	green and sweet	
Millet	Nuts	
Sardines	Oats	
Tofu	Onion	
Watermelons	Peanuts	
	Pumpkin	
	Rye	
	Sesame	
	Soybeans	
	Squash	
	Sunflower	
	Turnips	

Some are acid promoting as well, so use them only in moderation or as an occasional treat.

If you sort out your symptoms and see that you are consistently developing symptoms of disordered energy of one direction or the other, it's a good indication to tip the diet a bit toward the compensating energy.

The Kidney and Deficiency

In its traditional form, TCM is a complete system of primary healthcare. Macrobiotics is essentially a form modified for the layperson for day-to-day use. The Chinese, famed for their pragmatic outlook, historically tended to postulate the presence of an organ and its relation to a physiological function even if they could not identify an actual anatomical structure that was proven to carry out that function. If they could perceive a physiological function, they then attempted to describe appropriate organs. Chinese names for organs that have been translated into English show metaphors based on the functions that happen to be associated with the organs, not the specific organ tissues as we know them from modern science.

Further, since they mostly used herbs and food as medicine, and herbs have broad, nutritive actions, the Chinese had generally little need to get very specific. The kidney is a great example. In TCM, the concept of "kidney" encompasses a lot more than the modern physiological idea of the specific kidney organ. It includes all the physiological functions that make up the urinary system and the endocrine system, especially the adrenal glands. It regulates the electrolyte balance of sodium and potassium. The kidney is of paramount importance in TCM, so much so that it is thought that the primary cause of disease is a weak inherited constitution, lowered immune function, and lack of essence, all tied in with kidney, as the home of "ancestral chi," the reserve qi supply, present from birth. The kidney is the root source for all the yin and yang in the body, and its job is to regulate all yin and yang throughout the entire body.

Water balance is easy to understand. However, in TCM the "kidney" also is involved with storing, maintaining, and regulating the body's vital energy. It is the reserve for stamina. The adrenal glands are attached to the tops of both kidneys. Though not strictly made of kidney tissue, they are in close proximity with the actual kidney organs, and TCM merges the two functions into one master concept. The focal point of Chinese physiological theory is function rather than form, so the TCM "kidney" concept gives a more holistic perspective in terms of its effect on the body and mind.

The kidney has yin and yang functions. Yin relates to the container that receives energy, and yang relates to the life energy that fills it. Yin qualities include substantial, cool, and moist. The kidney is connected with physiological functions that are cooling, receptive, tissue building, and sustaining. Yang represents ephemeral, warm, mobile, and dry. It is warming, aggressive, tissue reducing, transforming, and protective.

The TCM concept of kidney yin very significantly involves the secretion of hormones, including cortisol, from the adrenal cortex. A yin deficiency means that the preserving and repairing function of the body is depleted or missing. Generally, in yin deficiency, yang chi overflows and creates an assortment of hypermetabolic signs, such as heat, nervousness, flushed complexion, chronic inflammation, and wasting. Specifically, deficient kidney yin creates symptoms of lumbar soreness, leg and knee weakness, tinnitus, feverish sensation in the soles and palms, nocturnal emission, and scanty menstrual flow. Yin is like the lubricating oil in your car engine. Without its lubrication, the engine parts grind themselves to pieces. In the body, arthritis, with painful, dry, twisted joints, is a good example of a yin deficiency disease.

All these yin deficiency symptoms are chronic and wasting in nature. In the West, we call this "burnout" or "adrenal fatigue." Many folks have an ongoing condition of stress-induced chronic yin deficiency. The body requires some amount of yang adrenaline to produce motivation to react to stress and to succeed in life, but it also has a practically constant need for cortisol to buffer that same stress.

Moist, soothing, nutritive foods, such as oatmeal, and herbs with these qualities, such as licorice, rebuild the deficient yin and treat the deficiency.

Kidney yang involves hormone secretions, including adrenaline, from the adrenal medulla. In general, a yang deficiency involves signs of coldness, paleness, fatigue, low libido, and edema. Specifically, kidney yang can involve fatigue, coldness, lack of libido, impotence, frequent clear urine, night urination, premature ejaculation, and edema of the lower limbs. Kidney yang deficiency can also involve retarded growth and sexual development and hair loss.

These concepts of yin and yang deficiency are critically important in TCM. Deficiency of yin or yang in the kidney is especially problematic, as the kidney is said to store and regulate all energy in the body. Therefore, we can have a problem of overabundant yang energy (hot, excited, intense) caused by too much yang, or the corresponding problem, often with similar symptoms, caused by deficient offsetting yin. As a parallel, we can have a problem of overabundant yin energy (wet, cold, passive) caused by too much yin, or the corresponding problem, often with similar symptoms, caused by deficient offsetting yang. In our culture, yin deficiency is extremely common, as our high stress level burns up our reserve of nourishing, lubricating, soothing yin juices.

According to Dr. Michael Tierra, "George Ohsawa was a Japanese-Chinese Medicine practitioner. When he brought macrobiotics to the West, he reversed the classification of Yin and Yang, which is a complicated issue, but essentially because he knew that the Western mind was not prepared to understand the dynamic nature of yin and yang theory and would have difficulty understanding the important Chinese Medical concept of Yin Deficiency." Macrobiotics presents yin and yang in a fairly straightforward way that people can grasp and use, but people may miss a lot of the subtlety of original TCM in the process, particularly the need to nourish yin. Macrobiotics posits a pretty clear-cut balance, where you balance one energy by consuming more of the other, rather than the possibility of nurturing the deficiency. Since the concept of yin deficiency is so descriptive of what most Americans have going on, it is a valuable concept to add to the basics of macrobiotics.

Acid and Alkaline in Macrobiotics

Herman Aihara was born in Japan in 1920. He studied with the founder of macrobiotics, George Ohsawa, before World War II. Eventually he emigrated to the United States to teach macrobiotics. He worked with the better-known macrobiotics proponent, Michio Kushi, in New York from 1952 to 1961. He founded the George Ohsawa Macrobiotic Foundation in San Francisco in 1974.

Aihara did extensive work in correlating the modern concepts of pH and the ancient ideas of Asian medicine as expressed in macrobiotics. Not satisfied to stop with calling yang "acid" and yin "alkaline," Aihara evaluated the content of acid- versus alkaline-forming minerals in foods that were known in macrobiotics to be yin or yang. For example, a meal of rice, fish, tofu, and beer, while well balanced between yin and yang, includes only acid foods. Aihara would suggest adding alkaline foods, such as radish and leafy greens.

Aihara looked at the content of alkaline minerals in foods. Calcium is alkalinizing, so Aihara suggested obtaining it in abundance from vegetables and seaweeds. We don't often eat turnip greens here, but they are a rich source of calcium. A cup of turnip greens contains 229 milligrams of calcium. You can steam them right along with the turnip roots. A sea vegetable that is very rich in calcium is hijiki, which contains 610 milligrams of calcium per cup. Rinse and soak dry hijiki for at least fifteen minutes before you use it. This seaweed is very tasty prepared with onion, tofu, carrots, sesame oil, and soy sauce. Aihara calculated that potassium, sodium, magnesium, and iron are also alkalinizing minerals, and again encouraged vegetables and seaweeds as sources.

Aihara also looked at the acid minerals in foods. Concerned about the formation of phosphoric acid from phosphorus in the diet, he cautioned against eating excessive phosphorus-containing foods. He taught that animal foods were too dominant in phosphorus to be suitable as proper food. Sulfur similarly forms sulfuric acid, so he didn't like sulfur much, either. Sulfur is common in the soil, but we don't eat many vegetables that are particularly abundant in sulfur to any great extent. The onion family, which also includes garlic, chives, and leeks, has a lot of sulfur, as does the cabbage family, whose members include broccoli, cauliflower, and kale. All these vegetables contain numerous other alkalinizing minerals, though, so the sulfur is probably not much of a concern.

In particular, Aihara focused on the ratio of calcium to phosphorus in foods. Since calcium is alkaline and phosphorus is acid, he postulated that foods with a high calcium content in relation to phosphorus are alkalinizing and better for most people. Hijiki, the Japanese seaweed mentioned above, has an extremely high ratio of more than twenty-five times as much calcium as phosphorus. Other foods with relatively high ratios are kombu and nori, which are also seaweeds, as well as green onions, spinach, sesame seeds, tofu, radishes, and tangerines. Bancha, a popular Asian tea made from the twigs, rather than the leaves, of the green tea bush, has a high calcium to phosphorus ratio of 3.6. Foods with abysmal calcium to phosphorus ratios include chicken, pork, tuna, white rice, and white bread.

Aihara cross-classified the pH of the mineral content of foods to the traditional macrobiotic classifications and came up with a fourfold scheme that he called "the four wheel balance of foods" (see Figure 4.1). We can see from Figure 4.1 that the correspondence was not always consistent, but that, on the whole, the system provides a target and a strategy for adjusting our diet when we know where we are on the yin-yang continuum and the pH continuum.

Asian healing systems disagree about how to approach table salt. That's because, as sodium chloride, it is a chemical combination of a strongly alkalinizing element, sodium, and a strongly acidifying element, chlorine. In the stomach, the chlorine tends to increase acidity, since stomach acid is hydrochloric acid. Ayurveda, as you recall, says that salt is warming, albeit only mildly.

TCM, in contrast, is more interested in the sodium content, which promotes water retention, thereby making tissues wetter. Water is cooling, hence the taste and temperature definition. Macrobiotics looks at the flip side. Since water swells tissue, making it thicker and more able to retain heat, Ohsawa called salty taste hot, in a minor break with TCM

Yin Acid-Forming Foods	Yin Alkaline-Forming Foods
Alcohol	Bancha tea
Beans and peas	Cocoa
Nuts	Coffee
Pharmaceutical drugs (most)	Cucumbers
Sugar	Dates
Tofu	Eggplants
Vinegar	Grapes
	Honey
	Lemons
	Mustard
	Potatoes
	Raisins
	Sesame seeds
	Sunflower seeds
	Vegetables
Yang Acid-Forming Foods	**Yang Alkaline-Forming Foods**
Animal foods	Dry radish pickles
Grains	Millet
	Miso
	Salt
	Salted umeboshi plums
	Soy sauce

Figure 4.1. The Four Wheel Balance of Foods

theory. According to Dr. Tierra, "from [Ohsawa's] perspective salt was important because it increased one's capacity to retain fluid which in turn would help the body to retain warmth." Most Americans are too cold and fatigued. Macrobiotics puts an emphasis on consuming plenty of salty taste.

People who have consumed a lot of meat for a long time tend to be full of acid. Macrobiotics sees acidosis, common to Americans, as the root of many different diseases, including diabetes, high blood pressure, and arthritis. They view it as being caused by acid-forming foods, anger, worry, fear, shallow breathing, and rarely, physical overwork. Enlarged pupils and crossed eyes are signs of acidosis.

Macrobiotics recommends beginning with a basic food program of alkaline-forming foods to begin the recovery from acidosis. If you start gradually and make only a few overall changes in your food selections at a time, you will achieve significant progress toward balancing the chemistry and energy of your body. You make additional refinements as you gain experience. Following are a few noted macrobiotic staple healing foods.

Miso is a product made by fermenting soy, closely related to the process used to produce the familiar soy sauce condiment. It is a salty paste that comes in many different colors and flavors, from dark brown and earthy to light yellow and mellow. Miso is rich in alkaline minerals. Use it as a savory base for broths and soups. It is about the consistency of peanut butter. Use about 1 teaspoon of miso for every cup of broth or soup and allow it to dissolve fully.

Wakame is a flat, salty seaweed that is popular in macrobiotic cooking. Like other sea vegetables, it is rich in minerals. It has a very respectable calcium-to-phosphorus ratio of 5. Buy dried wakame and soak it in water until it softens up. Like all seaweeds, it has a salty taste. Add wakame as a vegetable ingredient to stews and casseroles. For a delicious, simple soup, add miso to water to your taste, add chopped softened wakame, and simmer, covered, until the wakame is tender. If desired, add a bit of sautéed onion. Tasty!

Aduki beans, sometimes called adzuki or azuki beans, are small Asian beans that pack a nutritional wallop. About the size of a small peanut, they are dark red and the shape of a kidney bean. A staple of macrobiotic healing diets, they make a complete protein when served with rice. Because aduki beans are so small, they cook up quickly without needing to be presoaked or pressure cooked. A bean from India, the mung bean, is very similar (except for the color) and can be used in a similar manner.

Daikon is a very large white radish that is ubiquitous in East Asian cooking. You might have enjoyed some daikon in your sushi or pickled as an appetizer at a Korean restaurant. You can steam daikon as a tasty vegetable much the same as you do carrots and turnips. One yummy style is simply to grate the radish, raw, onto grains or into soup.

Cucumbers are also preferred in macrobiotics for alkalinizing. In Asia, this popular vegetable is served in many ways, from fresh in sushi or as a side dish, to pickled as a condiment. Other popular vegetables are cabbage, which is preserved in brine and added to the alkalinizing diet, and spinach, another alkalinizing green vegetable commonly found in macrobiotic recipes. Boiled, spinach is eaten as a simple side dish.

One very famous food that has become popular in macrobiotics is salted umeboshi plum. This fruit, a plum about the size of a cherry, is very tart from natural acids. It is dried and preserved in salt. A very yang food, it is nevertheless alkalinizing, according to Aihara. Pop one in your mouth and suck on the salty flesh as a digestive aid or swallow one or two before a meal to stimulate digestive juices.

Alkalosis, on the other hand, is evidenced by overreaction, lack of emotion, contracted pupils, and eyes that drift outward (wall eyes). Alkalosis is adjusted by upping the proportion of whole grains, which are slightly acid forming, in the diet, and by chewing the food more thoroughly.[1] You could theoretically use acid foods such as red meat to balance this condition, but such an approach is extreme and seen as unnecessary in macrobiotics.

Macrobiotic living has millions of adherents around the world. The diet is famous in some quarters for reducing cancer. Easy to use, it is a scheme that makes good sense, as do all the older holistic systems. People find their diet empowering, and there is no doubt that the emphasis on healthy food and lifestyle is quite beneficial. By combining the ideas of yin and yang with a more modern understanding of pH, Mr. Aihara has expanded an already effective system, giving it another dimension that goes one level deeper to help manage health. Even a few of these simple changes can make a big difference.

5

Health and Disease in Asian Healing

We've talked a lot about the theory of body balance. But can real people put these ideas into practice? It just takes doing it. Several modern health authorities have established programs that utilize these practices in a daily routine that assists sick people with becoming well and healthy people with getting even better. And you can apply their discoveries in your daily life. Let's see how they did it.

Cleansing and Balancing pH Helps Healing

Kartar Singh Khalsa, D.O.M., combines the expertise of a licensed doctor of Oriental medicine, a trained acupuncturist, and a kundalini yoga teacher. He currently maintains a private practice in northern New Mexico, where he employs herbalism and acupuncture to treat his patients. He has designed a detoxifying program based on alkalinizing the body. Over the last five years, Dr. Khalsa has guided more than 1,000 people through the New Cleanse, as well as participated in the program more than twenty-five times himself.

The New Cleanse is a ten-day program featuring a collection of 100-percent vegan Chinese herbs, Ayurvedic herbs, and nutritional supplements. The New Cleanse also uses detoxifying and strengthening methods to reestablish the body's integrity at a cellular level.

As clinical director of his facility, Dr. Khalsa is responsible for coordinating case management for the numerous patients. His colleagues at the facility include a chiropractor, a medical doctor, and several holistic therapists of various types.

Dr. Khalsa says that alkalinity is currently an important factor because many people in our culture have lifestyle habits that create a more acidic environment. Coffee, carbonated soft drinks, fast food, and toxins in general all have acidic natures. He has found in his practice that the more people smoke, drink alcohol, overeat, or eat unhealthy foods, the more acidic they are. Medical doctors aren't trained to look at pH levels unless the levels become life threatening, so they often overlook pH. The pH is an important consideration in returning the body to its original balance. An acidic pH puts a strain on the body as it works to return to balance, and it robs the body of vitamins and minerals, particularly trace minerals, as it struggles to maintain optimum pH.

Dr. Khalsa measures the pH of the body using urine strips. He can usually correct pH imbalance with diet, using fresh foods of an alkaline nature. He also incorporates yoga and meditation to balance pH.

Enzymes are involved in every metabolic process. Our immune system, bloodstream, liver, kidneys, spleen, and pancreas, as well as our abilities to see, think, and breathe, depend on enzymes. Enzymes initiate all cellular activity. Enzymes break down toxic substances so that the body can eliminate them without damaging the eliminative organs. It is in our best interest always to have plenty of enzyme reserves. The New Cleanse program finds this to be very important. Unfortunately, enzymes are destroyed at approximately 120 degrees Fahrenheit. Therefore, it is best to take supplemental enzymes if you cook your foods.[1]

Theodore A. Baroody, D.C., N.D., Ph.D., C.N.C., is a practitioner specializing in pH-balancing therapies. He is the author of the forcefully titled *Alkalize or Die* (Holographic Health, 1991). He has created an entire program of diet and supplementation. Dr. Baroody's ideas are a bit unorthodox, even for the alternative health world. As you can see from the title of his book, his methods are very direct. Nonetheless, many professionals applaud his methods. Dr. Khalsa is especially impressed with Dr. Baroody's theories and bases some of the techniques he uses in the New Cleanse on Dr. Baroody's work.

Normal life stresses organ systems. Cleansing and detoxification begin the process of rehabilitation of the organ systems. Cleansing and detoxification are ancient and transformational endeavors that have been practiced for thousands of years by many different cultures.

The New Cleanse uses detoxifying and strengthening methods to reestablish the body's balanced chemistry. The New Cleanse begins with diet. A simple but specific alkaline diet nourishes the body with a nutritionally balanced combination of foods and grains.

Kundalini yoga exercises encourage breath—the life source of the body—and help to stimulate and assist the functions of the lymph system and the nervous system. Specific daily Kundalini yoga sets are included in the New Cleanse to facilitate the detoxification process and to support the participants while they move through the different phases of the program.

During the ten-day process, colon and liver cleansing helps to remove toxins and parasites. Chemicals, heavy metals, and other toxins are eliminated from the liver to restore both physical and mental balance. Parasites, viruses, yeasts, and bacteria are released from the colon, giving participants the ability to benefit more fully from the nutrition in the foods they eat.

The primary tools used, however, are diet, herbs, and supplements. Current thinking is to create an alkaline environment using fresh fruits and vegetables. Supplements, herbs, micronutrients, and trace minerals give the body what it needs when going through this process of cleansing and detox. Ayurvedic and Chinese herbs support the organ systems that are stressed.

Dr. Khalsa relies on a finely tuned selection of supplements in his private practice and in the New Cleanse. To alkalinize the body, Dr. Khalsa favors a program containing:

- High-potency proteolytic digestive enzymes (protease, amylase, lipase, trypsin, papain, bromelain, lysozyme, and chymotrypsin in a base of a special bicarbonate complex)
- Essential fatty acids
- Calcium, in the form of 2-aminoethyl phosphate (calcium EAP)
- Acidophilus
- Magnesium oxide
- Selected Chinese and Ayurvedic herbs (including bhumy amalaki, amla fruit, cinchona bark, pau d'arco bark, black pepper, thyme leaf, and yucca root)

The New Cleanse uses bhumy amalaki to promote healthy liver function and to provide general liver support. This herb is the main general liver herb of Ayurveda. The New Cleanse also uses Colosan, a form of magnesium oxide, to restore colon hygiene by eliminating built-up toxins before providing the body with what it needs to restore well-being and rejuvenation. According to the folks at the New Cleanse, there is no better way to clean the colon than with oxygen, since digestion is a process of oxidation. By introducing oxygen into the intestines and the colon through the use of Colosan, we can assist the process of complete digestion as well as of oxidizing undigested material. Colosan turns undigested material in the intestines into carbon dioxide, waste, and water. It is very logical to clean out the organs of elimination prior to attempting to detoxify the body. This way the body can eliminate the toxins more readily rather than have them stirred up and floating around. Common symptoms of a healing crisis are nausea, headache, tiredness, and pain in the liver and kidney areas. By cleaning out the organs of elimination through the use of Colosan, detox reactions—that is, healing crises associated with cleansing programs—can be avoided or minimized.

Dr. Khalsa says that "Colosan enables a cleansing of all twenty-one feet of the digestive tract as well as loosening the impacted material in the lower colon. The goal is to clear the small intestine and colon of congested material and improve their functions of assimilation, absorption, and elimination. The average person has a certain amount of accumulated waste in the gut. Your body mixes these materials in mucus to keep itself from being irritated. This is a resting ground for parasites, germs, bacteria and viruses."

The New Cleanse also uses Digeplex, a combination of gentian root, goldenseal root, clove bud, papaya leaf, ginger root, and turmeric root, to offer general support to the gastrointestinal tract. Turmeric root is well known for its astringent and anti-inflammatory qualities. Free radicals are normally produced when chemical reactions occur in the body, and even more free radicals can be produced during times of stress, such as during cleansing and detoxification. Antioxidants are used to give the body support for the naturally occurring chemical reactions. Antioxidants include vitamins A, C, and E and the mineral selenium.

Dr. Khalsa additionally relies on amla, the main rejuvenative herb of Ayurveda. Amla is believed to have the highest content of vitamin C in the plant world and is therefore a very potent antioxidant. Triphala, the most famous Ayurvedic formula, includes amla fruit as a part of its formula. Triphala is a very general rejuvenative formula. Known primarily as an antioxidant, it also supports the endocrine system, the skin, the eyes, and the liver. Used over time, triphala promotes stamina, hormone balance, and regularity. It fights aging, particularly of the skin, as well as loss of visual acuity associated with aging.

Body Balancing the Chinese Way

In TCM, there is a concept of inherent potential energy, or original, ancestral qi, which is inherited from parents and resides in the kidneys. The primal spark of life, it cannot be increased or restored by food herbs, water, or air. The only way it can be increased is through intensive meditation practices, but most Americans do not have time for these. We can therefore expect to live a life with a finite amount of kidney essence. Consumed over a lifetime, it gradually results in the process of aging, decline, and death.

Chinese medicine uses many techniques to heal, but primarily it is a system of herbal medicine and therapeutic diet. TCM has been around for a long time, and Chinese healers have developed uses for about 6,000 different species of herbs. Some of these herbs truly stand out. TCM has a category of "superior medicines." These are medicines that have an effect over the long term, are nutritive and foodlike in character, affect multiple systems, increase stamina and immune function, and are usually taken in modest doses over a span of many years. Often these herbs are called "tonics." In the TCM scheme, they support the kidney, the source of stamina. They are the ultimate Asian body-balancing therapies.

Licorice root (*Glycyrrhiza uralensis*) is the classic example of such an herb. This herb, which is drastically sweet in taste, is called the "universal harmonizer" in Chinese medicine. It is believed to enhance the actions of other herbs in a formula and to ameliorate any undesirable reaction to any single herb or combination of other herbs in a prescription. Licorice appears in virtually every Chinese formula and is the most commonly prescribed Chinese herb. It improves the flavor of Chinese teas, which are renowned for their bad taste. Licorice has the advantage of being neutral in temperature, so it is suitable for almost everyone.

TCM classifies licorice as a tonic for qi. It is a tissue-moistening herb, so it supports the nourishing yin energy in the body. It is also used for pain, coughs, irritated and inflamed tissues, allergies, and colds.

Licorice has cortisone-like action. Glycyrrhizin, the main active constituent, is chemically similar to certain adrenal cortical hormones, including cortisol. In the bloodstream, licorice can mimic the action of these hormones and works at least in part by extending the time that corticoid hormones remain active. Because of this action, licorice has noted anti-inflammatory powers. With its soothing cortisol action, it reduces the possibility of any irritating actions from other herbs, "softening" their curative effects.

People of southern Europe use a closely related species (*Glycyrrhiza glabra*) as a cough and mucus-loosening remedy. Quite by chance, European pharmacists investigating the respiratory actions of this licorice stumbled on its effectiveness in the treatment of gastric ulcers. Like cortisone and other anti-inflammatory medicines, licorice inhibits inflammatory reactions and can relieve the symptoms of peptic ulcers.

Excess long-term licorice use can produce edema, just like the drug cortisone does. TCM would call that imbalance "deficient kidney yang." As with the drug therapy, licorice taken in sustained high doses can cause elevated potassium levels and hypertension. Don't use licorice if you have a tendency toward renal hypertension.

Licorice is not appropriate for people with excess yin, especially if they have bloating, edema, and renal hypertension. Women are more yin by nature and have an even stronger propensity for fluid retention. Therefore, licorice is used conservatively in women's formulas—no more than 12 grams per day—because of the hormone mimic effects, but that is usually not an issue, as licorice is mildly stool loosening, so most folks can't tolerate 12 grams per day anyway.

Di huang (*Rehmannia glutinosa*), another noted TCM root, is sometimes called Chinese foxglove. Like licorice, rehmannia contains a number of plant hormone compounds, including beta-sitosterol. Cured by soaking and drying the compressed roots nine times in rice wine, it is used as a nourishing blood and yin tonic. Rehmannia prepared this way is an important herb to nourish the blood and kidney yin. With kidney yang herbs, it supports kidney yang function.

Prepared rehmannia is used in the treatment of anemia, often with another famous TCM blood builder, dong quai. With dong quai, it also is employed for yin dizziness, tinnitus, weakness, pain of the lower back and legs, and amenorrhea. This famous herb also benefits the immune system by stimulating red blood cell formation in the bone marrow. Rehmannia also helps the liver dispense with aged red blood cells.

Use rehmannia in a dose of 10 grams per day to nourish, tonify, and harmonize the body and to build new healthy blood.

Siberian ginseng (*Eleutherococcus senticosus*) has been famous as a tonic herb. It is in the Araliaceae family, related to Panax ginseng. Its Chinese name is *ci wu jia*. This herb is not ginseng, although it is related. It does not grow in Siberia, but it is the main tonic herb of Siberia, just as Panax ginseng is the main tonic of East Asia. Many practitioners prefer to call this herb eleuthero root to distinguish it from true ginseng.

Eleuthero has a mildly warming energy, so it is not as appropriate for yin deficiency or hot conditions. Eleuthero is more of a warming kidney yang tonic with some of the cortisol anti-inflammatory effects. Paradoxically, this herb also is used in TCM as a slow-acting anti-inflammatory in arthritis. As is typical with these slow-acting tonic herbs and foods, eleuthero responds appropriately to the needs of the body, warming and stimulating or cooling and sedating as necessary for the individual.

Eleuthero has been extensively researched by Russian scientists. It has become popular around the world to improve performance and endurance.

Schisandra (*Schisandra chinensis*) is an East Asian woody vine in the Magnolia family. Winding around the trunks of trees, and covering their branches, the vine produces small red berries that grow in clusters. In the fall, the berries are harvested and dried to make the medicinal herb.

The Chinese name for this herb is *wu wei tze*, or "five-flavor berry," indicating that the fruit contains all five flavors of the Chinese herbal pharmacy. Herbs with this taste profile are rare, and this detail predicts schisandra's use in a wide variety of conditions. Schisandra is mostly sour, though, and most definitely astringent.

In Asian medicine, schisandra is essentially a general tonic, used to "prolong the years of life without aging," a sort of "poor man's ginseng." Traditionally, hunters and athletes have used schisandra with the conviction that it will increase endurance and fight fatigue under physical stress. It is also used as a male sexual tonic.

Russian and Chinese traditional medicine has long used schisandra for a wide variety of conditions, including coughs and other respiratory ailments, diarrhea, insomnia, impotence, and kidney problems. Chinese medicine considers it specific for asthma. According to Asian medicine, it regulates blood circulation, blood sugar, blood pressure, and heart rhythm.

Schisandra seeds contain lignans, which are believed to be active constituents. Modern Chinese research suggests that these lignans stimulate the immune system, protect the liver, increase stress coping, and may produce a mild sedative effect. The main lignans in schisandra are schizandrin, wuweizisu C, and gomisin A.

The most promising area in which schisandra berry is used, however, is in treating liver damage in conditions such as hepatitis. In China, schisandra berries are widely used for progressive hepatic degeneration due to viral hepatitis or chemical damage. Recently, numerous animal studies have indicated that schisandra berry protects the liver from damage.

Most physicians who practice traditional herbal medicine in Japan have observed that schisandra can be as effective as interferon therapy in the treatment of chronic hepatitis C. A 2000 Japanese study determined that an herbal compound containing schisandra was particularly effective and that this herb was the most potent ingredient. It was further determined that the benefit was due to a suppression of the hepatitis C virus.

The astringent qualities of the schisandra berry make it ideal for what the Chinese call "preserving the essence"—that is, keeping leaking fluids retained where they belong. Used predominantly for the lungs and kidneys to arrest mucous discharges, schisandra is therefore excellent for bed-wetting, urinary incontinence, postnasal drip, and spermatorrhea, the involuntary loss of semen. In my experience as a clinical herbalist, this remedy is especially effective for night sweats.

Schisandra berries actually taste good, so they can be taken as a tea or even cooked into food such as soup broth. This herb is quite mild and foodlike, so feel free to use as much as you care to. Use a high dose acutely, then a small daily dose for maintenance. The TCM dose is 10 grams per day in food or tea. Remember that the effects are slow and gradual, and extend over a period of years.

These time-honored berries have been used in folk medicine for a variety of complaints that plague us daily. They make a good-tasting tea and food, and are safe for just about anyone to use. Add them to your life, and you will have another pillar for your health program.

He shou wu root (*Polygonum multiflorum*) is native to China, where it continues to be widely grown. Here, it is often incorrectly called fo-ti, a fanciful name that is not correct in Chinese. (However, the misnomer is so common that Chinese herb stores recognize it.) Once it has been boiled in a special black bean liquid, it is considered a superior medicine according to TCM. The Chinese common name, *he shou wu*, is from the name of a famous herbalist whose infertility was supposedly cured by the herb. In addition, the herbalist's long life was credited to the tonic properties of this herb. TCM uses fo-ti to treat premature aging, weakness, vaginal discharges, numerous infectious diseases, angina pectoris, premature hair loss and graying, and impotence, all signs of kidney yin deficiency, or adrenal depletion. (The name translates as "Mr. He's black hair.") He shou wu is also well suited to tonifying the thyroid.

The active constituents of he shou wu have yet to be determined. The whole root has been shown to lower cholesterol levels, according to animal and human research, as well as to decrease atherosclerosis. Other research has investigated this herb's role in strong immune function, red blood cell formation, and antibacterial action. The roots have a mild laxative action.

Use up to 15 grams of dried he shou wu per day in capsules or as tea. The tea has a pleasant earthy flavor that many people like as a coffee substitute. The chopped herb can be brewed like coffee. Since he shou wu is a nutritive tonic herb, it is common in TCM to take it for years at a time. It should be available in your nearby herb store.

One of the most popular and effective forms of he shou wu is in a Chinese formula product called Shou Wou Chih. A liquid extract containing he shou wu, dong quai, ligusticum, polygonatum, and rehmannia root, Shou Wou Chih aids circulation and digestion. As a liver and kidney tonic, it tonifies, warms, and invigorates the blood. It is widely used to strengthen the eyes, bones, and tendons of the back, and to relieve joint pains and disorders caused by the depleting circumstances of excess sexual activity, childbirth, or illness. Shou Wou Chih is often taken daily for many months at a dose of 2 to 3 tablespoons three times a day.

Black sesame seeds are revered in TCM and Ayurveda. Black sesame is an oil-rich food that increases physical and sexual stamina and promotes the growth and health of the hair.

A good long-term maintenance dose is 1 tablespoon per day. Ayurveda uses a drink made by combining 1 tablespoon of ground black sesame seed with 10 ounces of warm milk, 1 tablespoon of ghee (clarified butter), and 1 teaspoon of honey as a sexual building remedy. Dry-roast and grind the seeds with a little salt to make a tasty condiment. Sprinkle the mixture on rice and other foods. He shou wu and black sesame work well together in a daily rejuvenation program.

The Kidneys and the Hair

Kidney qi is the fount of stamina for the whole body. It is manifested obviously in the hair. When it is vital and abundant, the hair is radiant, full of color, and lustrous. If kidney qi declines, the hair loses its color, withers, and drops out. Since aging is measured by the decline in kidney energy, hair changes are inevitable. People with a deficiency of kidney yin will tend toward hair graying. The TCM internal medicine treatment for hair loss is to nourish both kidney yin and yang. This approach will strengthen the autonomic nervous system and the endocrine system. Use kidney tonic herbs, especially he shou wu and rehmannia, to keep your hair strong and healthy.

Asian healing defines health as balance. Over the thousands of years that folks have been applying these principles, they have learned an awful lot about what makes people tick. Our ancestors figured out, through generations of careful observation, what puts people out of balance and how to remedy that by using herbs, foods, and lifestyle changes to nudge the body's energies back into place.

In our busy modern lives, we have considerable trouble staying balanced, so these ideas are even more important. I have seen these principles become lifesaving additions to people's routines. They work, and they work well. It may take a bit of effort to get started with these new medicines and foods, but the results are truly striking. Simple things such as having some black sesame ready for seasoning the dinner, or brewing a cup of tea from he shou wu, or cooking some schisandra berries into your rice can make very nice changes over time. Start with one or two of these notions, then add more practices as you go. Very small course corrections, started now, can lead to a completely new destination fifty years in the future. And you know those fifty years will pass anyway, so you might as well arrive at your destination a bit healthier and happier.

6

Body Balance in Naturopathy

The term "naturopathy" was coined in the United States at the beginning of the twentieth century. But the philosophy on which naturopathy is based has been universally used to treat diseases since ancient times. Hippocrates taught that "nature is healer of all diseases." He articulated the concept *vis medicatrix naturae* ("the healing power of nature"), which has long been at the heart of indigenous medicine in many cultures around the world and is at the core of naturopathic medicine. The earliest healers toiled with food, herbs, water therapies, fasting, detoxification, and tissue manipulation. These gentle treatments work along with the body's own healing powers. Contemporary naturopathic physicians carry on these therapies as their main tools. They also advocate prevention as a mainstay of good health.

Natural medicine was popular and widely available in the United States well into the early part of the twentieth century. But the rise of conventional, drug-and-surgery-based medicine, along with the discovery and increasing use of miracle drugs such as antibiotics, by mid-century caused a temporary decline of naturopathy and most other systems of natural healing. By the 1970s, American consumers were becoming increasingly disenchanted with conventional medicine, and millions were inspired to look for alternatives. Naturopathy and complementary alternative medicine entered a renaissance.

Naturopathy, now more often called "naturopathic medicine," is a modern holistic health approach that combines traditional healing techniques with the latest discoveries in biochemical sciences. In the United States, the profession's organization and functioning include accrediting educational institutions, licensing practitioners, formulating comprehensive standards of practice, peer review, and serious commitment to state-of-the-art scientific research. American naturopathic physicians hold the N.D. degree. They employ therapies that are primarily natural and nontoxic, among them clinical nutrition, homeopathy, herbal medicine, hydrotherapy, manipulative therapies, and counseling. Naturopathic physicians may also have additional training in specialties such as acupuncture and home birthing. These modern-day naturopathic physicians practice as primary healthcare providers.

Naturopathic medicine is identified by its fundamental principles of prevention; gentle, nontoxic therapies; and the healing power of nature. Within that scope, there is wide latitude for specific therapies and methods, depending on the needs of the patient. The practices include clinical and laboratory diagnostic testing, including diagnostic radiology and other imaging techniques; supplemental nutrients; therapeutic diets; fasting; natural medicinal substances, including herbs; hygiene; homeopathy; acupuncture; psychotherapy; minor surgery; natural childbirth; manipulative therapies; hydrotherapies; heat; cold; ultrasound; and therapeutic exercise. Naturopathic practice does not include major surgery or synthetic drugs.

For many diseases, naturopathic treatments can be primary and even curative. Naturopathic physicians offer the best in complementary medicine and cooperate with conventional medical practitioners when necessary. Modern naturopathy is a wide-ranging profession with a large collection of diagnostic techniques and a large palette of possible therapies. Any given naturopathic physician may or may not use any given technique. But one thing they all agree on: Keeping the body chemistry in balance is an important goal.

Explicitly or implicitly, many of the basic tenets of naturopathy are consistent with the modern ideas of pH balance. Among the proponents of pH-balancing schemes are naturopathic physicians or physicians with related credentials and holistic leanings. While pH measurement and adjustment, as such, are still somewhat out of the mainstream of contemporary naturopathy, if there is such a thing, they are gaining momentum in this profession, as they are in the ranks of orthodox medical professionals.

Detoxification

Naturopathic medicine has a core concept that is fundamental to success in almost all therapies. Naturopathic physicians are very interested in making sure that the body completely eliminates its metabolic wastes, which are all highly acidic, and that new damaging substances do not enter the body and wreak havoc. Prevention and clean living are of course primary, but what can you do if the damage is already done and the body is stuffed with noxious molecules? You can detoxify.

The body needs to get rid of its waste products to avoid becoming awash in its own wastes. When the body is burdened with harmful materials, normal physiological functions can become seriously disrupted, leading to chronic illness. Furthermore, the body's ability to absorb and distribute nutrients becomes severely limited. Because of its disrupted physiological processes and poor nutritional state, the body's ability to heal itself is severely degraded.

Unfortunately, the natural healing concept of detoxification is hard to define. The traditional idea is metaphorical, not a well-defined process of physiology. What we can say is that the signs of a need to detoxify are well known, the practical process of "detoxification" is well understood, we know when it has been accomplished because the signs go away, people feel a lot better after being "detoxified," and on the whole, clinical and laboratory signs of disease improve with the process.

First, let's define a few important terms. A "toxin" is a poisonous chemical that is produced by the metabolic activities of a plant or animal, unstable, causes damage when introduced into the tissues, and often stimulates antibody formation. Bee venom is a good example of a toxin. "Toxicity" is the presence of undesirable material in the body (from the natural healing point of view).

There is already a problem with the terms used in natural healing to describe this area. Physiologists use the label "toxin" in a very specific way. The natural healing use of the term, a much broader concept, is confusing to orthodox scientists. Functionally, we can say that poor digestion, colon sluggishness and dysfunction, reduced liver function, and poor elimination through the kidneys, respiratory tract, and skin all add to "toxicity," the buildup of excess undesirable materials in the tissues.

But just what is this material that collects to gum up the metabolic processes in the body? Just about anything that should not have been there in the first place, or an accumulation of normal body substances that haven't been eliminated. Broadly, we can divide these materials into two categories. "Endogenous toxins" are normal waste products that the body has not been able to eliminate adequately. Our bodies create these types of toxins in the process of normal functioning. Uric acid, a by-product of muscular effort, is an example. But one way or another, these substances must be neutralized or eliminated. If they are not, the consequences can include irritation and inflammation of our tissues, which jam normal functioning. The body, when functioning properly, is able to handle some toxicity, but it can become overwhelmed due to our poor habits and overexposure to these nasty wastes.

Toxicity has become of much greater concern in the twenty-first century than it has been at any time in the past. Until recently, most of the many thousands of chemicals to which we are exposed did not even exist. Our air, soil, and water are becoming increasingly saturated with this pollution. This exposure, along with our common use of drugs and refined foods, lack of exercise, and failure to drink enough water, has made us into toxic storehouses. "Exogenous toxins," the second category of toxins, are from the outside. Environmental pollutants such as the lead that remains from our previous widespread use of leaded gasoline and mercury from fish are good examples.

Lipids tend to be stored in the body, so body fat is also an accumulated adverse substance. Body fat tends to be a storage depot for fat-soluble poisons, such as dichlorodiphenyltrichloroethane (DDT). The more fat, the more storage! Arterial plaque and fatty lipomas (benign fatty tumors) are other examples. Remember that fat is essentially acid in pH by its nature.

Fluids can congregate where they don't belong. Edema, eye bags, and fluid-filled cysts are inappropriate collections of fluid that often contain high concentrations of damaging waste molecules. Blood can collect in stagnant areas, where it impedes the smooth movement of normal body fluids. Bruises, blood clots, and blood congested in the endometrium are good examples of congested blood. Minerals, even normal ones, can accumulate and, if present in excess, can cause problems. A bone spur is an example of an unhealthy mineral deposit. Toxic minerals such as lead and cadmium are damaging when they accumulate. Microbial by-products can be negative. Yeast, a normal inhabitant of the colon in appropriate numbers, produces alcohol as a normal by-product of its own metabolism. We all absorb small amounts of alcohol from our own intestinal yeast as a matter of course. But when the yeast reaches excess proportion, the alcohol can have an impact on our normal metabolism.

Normal body chemicals in excess can be a problem. Glucose, our normal blood sugar, causes diabetes when it's too high. Everyone has heard of the horrible consequences when that happens. So we can "detoxify" the excess glucose by making efforts to remove it. Even normal body wastes can become problematic if they accumulate in excess. If urine concentrates in the bladder, it can irritate and weaken the bladder tissue. Even constipation can be considered a type of toxicity.

So-called exogenous materials, substances that are not found naturally in the human body at all, can gather in the tissues. Petroleum-based chemicals, synthetic pesticides (such as DDT), dyes, and chemical additives from paint, cloth, carpeting, and other sources saturate our world in mind-boggling profusion. Most of these substances are fat soluble, so they become trapped in our fatty tissues and can remain stuck there for a lifetime.

Xenoestrogens are chemicals that mimic the action of estrogen in the body. They are often found in plastics and insecticides. As the world becomes more inundated with these chemicals, it is becoming obvious that they are causing insidious problems. Acting like hormones, they affect fundamental body systems, often disrupting fertility and sexual development.

Most of these stored substances are acid in pH or, at least, contribute to an acid condition. Only when all this gunk is removed from the tissues can the body function the way it was designed to, and you can go on to heal and excel in your life. Anything that supports elimination, from the micro level in the cells to the macro level in whole body systems, can be said to help us detoxify. The alternative medicine concepts of congestion, stagnation, and toxicity are closely interrelated. Detoxification is the process of clearing toxins from the body, or neutralizing or transforming them, and clearing excess mucus and congestion.

Detoxifying the body is frequently the first phase of natural therapeutic work. It is often seen as central in the treatment of chronic, degenerative diseases. A detoxification program can involve the use of homeopathic medicines, targeted dietary changes, nutritional supplements, and lymph stimulation therapies that focus on the elimination of toxins and waste products from the body at the cellular level.

Signs of the Need for Detoxification

So, how do you know that you need to be detoxified? Well, it's a safe bet that if you live in an industrialized society, you do. Since toxicity is at the root of nearly all chronic conditions, the symptoms are so common that they seem vague. Nonetheless, when you engage in some of these therapies and see the results, you will see for yourself that these lifelong signs, so normal for most of us, really can disappear. Consider yourself "toxic" if you have fatigue, swelling (eye bags, prostatitis), masses (cysts, fibroids, stones, clots), edema, headache, joint pain (and much other chronic pain), foul odor in general (stool, breath, perspiration), constipation (regularity or transit time), tissue discolorations (yellow skin, purple lips, brown mucus), tongue coating, discolored sclera (yellow or brown in the "white" of the eye), excess mucus (in the lungs or sinuses or in the stool), concentrated urine, conditions caused by natural chemical accumulations (gout), or skin disorders, especially inflammation (eczema, acne).

Detoxification Organs

After food is broken down in the stomach and small intestine and absorbed into the bloodstream, the nutrient constituents travel first to the liver. First and foremost, the liver modifies any toxic substances, making them water soluble so that they may pass easily from the body through the kidneys, or dissolving them in bile to be eliminated in the feces. If the liver fails, these damaging substances (from inside and outside the body) may accumulate, perhaps in the nervous and fatty tissues. According to natural healing practitioners, these "toxic" accumulations may contribute to Alzheimer's disease, Parkinson's disease, chronic fatigue syndrome, food and chemical allergies, headaches, hepatitis, and premenstrual syndrome. A main focus of naturopathic detoxification routines is getting the liver up to snuff with targeted food and herbal medicines. This is to increase blood flow through the liver, speeding the chemical reactions there and boosting the production of critical liver enzymes.

Next in importance is the large intestine. There is a saying in naturopathy that "all disease begins and ends in the colon." While this is certainly too general to be literally true, it comes close. The large intestine is the sewer for the body. Yet, when it is burdened by excess waste content, certain undesirable substances can be reabsorbed, only to be cycled yet again. Detoxification regimes often concentrate largely on enhancing colon function. They promote colon emptying by speeding transit time.

The kidney is the outlet for water-soluble wastes. As we have seen, it is also a serious dump for acid produced by normal body processes. While the kidneys have solid reserve capacity and usually work pretty well for a lifetime, they must be kept in good repair. Detoxification programs such as the New Cleanse typically use diuretic herbs to hasten the removal of water-soluble wastes from the tissues through the kidneys.

As we have seen, the skin and lungs do eliminate some wastes, including a bit of gas (from the lungs) that would otherwise contribute to the body's acid load. But they are not truly waste-removal organs. As backup routes out of the body, they can be emergency mechanisms, but the outgoing wastes tend to be tough on the delicate membrane tissues of these organs. Natural healing says that inflammatory skin diseases such as acne and eczema are the result of the body attempting to eliminate wastes through the skin, and we all can see the messes that result. Detoxification protocols that stimulate skin and lung elimination may work a little faster, but they usually end up making the person pretty uncomfortable in the meantime.

Detoxification Methods

One way or another, we can get all the eliminative channels cleaned out. Aerobic exercise increases circulation, boosts metabolic rate, and stimulates the exit of body by-products. We can also eject these materials more directly by using the body's own expulsion mechanisms: purging, diuresis, diaphoresis, expectoration, vomiting, all of which propel wastes out with immediacy. These direct methods tend to be less popular with Americans, as you can imagine. Chemical methods can work to zap toxins at the cellular level. Various nutrients and drugs will have effects for removing certain substances. Sulfur, zinc, copper, niacin, and antioxidants, including vitamins E and C, have detoxification action.

As for dietary adjustments, they can be very effective. Since food is less concentrated, it is a more diligent approach. Although it works well and is popular in many older systems, particularly in Ayurveda, modern Americans often find it tiresome and end up falling off the detox wagon before finishing the job. Detoxification diets feature food that is more digestible, with a lower calorie count. (Interestingly, people with heavy metal toxicity often do better with a high-protein, low-carbohydrate, no-grain diet, say naturopaths.)

Generally, the body goes through cycles of food processing (usually during the day) and detoxification (usually during the night). When the body does not get food for a while, it goes into detoxifying mode. That's the theory behind fasting. Temporarily reducing calorie intake, to whatever degree, will speed up detoxification. Upping water intake promotes fluid exchange and urination, so many experts recommend substantial water consumption while detoxifying. Heat increases circulation and urination, so crank up the sauna!

Naturopathic Protocols with pH

The Analyst is a service that provides naturopathic consultations online at digitalnaturopath.com. Designed and administered by naturopaths, it provides an expert system that generates an in-depth evaluation of a patient's health. Using a very detailed nine-page questionnaire, which takes between one-half and two hours to complete, the system gathers information about lifestyle habits, symptoms, vital statistics, and medical history. By using a combination of conventional Western medicine diagnostic techniques and the best of natural therapies, *The Analyst* addresses a long list of health problems, acute and chronic.

Responses to the multiple-choice questionnaire are translated into a health analysis that is based on statistical probabilities. The analysis is used to identify conditions that are likely to require attention and those that should be ruled out. The program also indicates treatments that have benefited previous patients with a similar profile. The service is valuable for physicians, who can tap into the large database of information. For patients, it provides the opportunity to benefit from the combined knowledge of more than one professional—that is, automatic second and third opinions. A person who wants to buy supplements at a health food store but needs advice on specifically which ones to pick can zero in on good possibilities. And for someone who is not easily able to visit a natural doctor, it is a good starting point. The computer-generated reports are reviewed by licensed naturopathic doctors who have attended four-year postgraduate medical schools. The report includes a summary of the reasoning behind the conclusions and suggestions provided.

The Analyst experts make the point that health problems rarely occur in isolation or for obvious reasons. That is exactly the idea behind understanding body chemistry. Based on the many signs the body gives, the experts propose that you can know what is *really* going on inside your body. These doctors agree that acidosis is an abnormality and that the naturopathic theory behind a correct dietary acid-alkaline balance is that because blood pH is slightly alkaline (usually falling within the range of 7.36 to 7.44), we should lean more toward eating alkaline foods. Naturopathically speaking, an acidic diet high in animal protein, sugar, caffeine, and processed foods tends to disrupt the pH balance. Depriving the body of alkaline minerals such as sodium, potassium, magnesium, and calcium leaves us prone to chronic and degenerative diseases. From this perspective, metabolic and respiratory acidosis are more extreme forms of pH imbalance, resulting from a variety of more serious disorders.

Based on naturopathic theory, there is a strong or generally accepted link among several signs, symptoms, and indicators that point toward acidosis. Among them are several that will already sound familiar. Allergy with excess mucus, congestion of the head and nose, frequent or severe colds and flus, and emotional irritability or anxiety are all indicative of acidosis. According to naturopathic physicians, if you have depression, increased osteoporosis symptoms or risk, general joint pain, muscle pain, neuritis, or neuropathy, there is a good chance that you are acidic. Based on current evidence, published in scientific journals, naturopathic theory supports the notion that acidic diets (high in protein and refined food) cause calcium to leach from bone in order to maintain blood pH balance, increasing the likelihood of osteoporosis. The same rationale implicates acidosis as a contributing cause in the development of neuritis.

Naturopathy highly recommends an alkalinizing diet for these conditions. Excluded in this scheme are foods that leave an acidic ash after being metabolized (proteins, starches, alcohol, and sugar). An alkaline diet is composed of approximately 75 percent alkaline foods and 25 percent acid foods, and includes low-acid fruits, vegetables, some fish and poultry, nuts and seeds, legumes, and whole grains. A healthy vegetarian diet may do some good.

Some naturopathic protocols add a few details for managing pH with a bit more finesse. Let's start with urine pH. If it's above 6.2, increase vitamin C, do not use vitamin D, and drink 1 teaspoon of apple cider vinegar in 4 ounces of water with each meal. If it's below 6.2, refrain from vitamin C, add vitamin D, and use ginger liberally as tea or a cooking herb.

Saliva pH is another story. If it's above 6.2, use kelp as a mineral source and take 2 tablespoons of olive oil per day as a bowel lubricant. If it's below 6.2, use a digestive enzyme with each meal, up your vitamin B_{12} dose, and include Coenzyme Q10. Also, blend a raw egg into 6 ounces of concord grape juice to assist your vitamin B_{12} uptake.

Naturopathic medicine is a wide and diverse discipline. Even so, at the core, there are some simple truths. By preventing disease, we will be a lot better off. If things do go astray, we can nudge the body and mind back into balance with gentle natural remedies. For hundreds of years, prominent naturopaths and their healer predecessors have lauded the value of moderation and balance. Now that more contemporary technical methods are available to assess what is going on in the tissues, we have one more lens through which to view the problem. This insight gives us great tools to apply to balancing body chemistry. As naturopathy continues to adopt the concepts of pH balance and to bring all their centuries of successful treatments to bear, the combination will be a powerful force for health and happiness.

7

What Science Has to Say

The term "pH" was coined in 1909. The "p" stands for *Potenz*, which is German for "power," and the "H" is the symbol for hydrogen.

The pH is a measurement scale that represents the relative concentration of hydrogen and hydroxyl ions in a liquid system. A hydrogen ion without its one electron is just a single proton, so pH is sometimes defined as proton concentration.

The pH of a substance is expressed on a scale of 0 to 14, with 0 signifying total hydrogen saturation and 14 total hydroxyl saturation. Distilled (pure) water is signified on the scale as neutral, with a pH of 7.0. Measurements of 6.9 down to 0.0 indicate acidity (more hydrogen ions), with the lower numbers being progressively more acidic. Measurements of 7.1 to 14.0 represent alkalinity (more hydroxyl ions), with the higher numbers being progressively more alkaline. For the pH of some common substances, see Table 7.1.

Substances can be referred to as neutral, acidic, or alkaline. The term "basic" means the same as alkaline.

The pH scale is logarithmic, like the Richter scale for earthquakes. Each unit of change on the scale represents a tenfold change in acidity or alkalinity. A solution with a pH of 1.0 is ten times more acidic than a solution with a pH of 2.0.[1]

The body responds to strong acids and strong bases with a sensation of burning. This is a result of the tissue damage caused by the chemical. Pure lye, for example, is strongly basic, with a pH of 13.0. If a drop gets on you when you are cleaning the bathroom, it is quite uncomfortable.

Table 7.1. The pH of Common Substances[2,3]	
Substance	**pH Level**
Hydrochloric acid	<1.0
Battery acid	1.0
Vinegar	2.4–3.4
Boric acid	5.0
Swimming pool water	7.4
Sea water	7.8–8.3
Baking soda (sodium bicarbonate)	8.3
Borax	9.3
Household ammonia	10.5–11.5
Lime (calcium hydroxide)	12.4
Milk of magnesia	12.5
Lye	13.0–13.6
Sodium hydroxide	14.0

And you can imagine what a drop of hydrochloric acid, with a pH of less than 1.0, would feel like on your skin.

The pH of Body Fluids

The stomach is the most acid spot in the entire body, with a pH of as low as 1.0. Stomach acid is very concentrated, and it forms the "acid reservoir" from which the body can draw if it needs to push down the pH of other fluids.

One of the ways the body can dump acid is releasing it into the urine. Depending on the total acid load in the body at any given time, the urine pH can be as acid as 4.5 to as mildly alkaline as 8.0.

The pH of the blood is controlled so tightly that the body does almost anything to keep it in the very narrow proper range of 7.30 to 7.45. You won't see much change here, even in the sickest patient.

The saliva is very slightly acidic.

The high concentrations of bicarbonate produced by the pancreas are secreted into the small intestine as part of the pancreatic digestive juices. This large bicarbonate store is the "alkaline reservoir." Bile, produced in the liver, stored in the gallbladder, and secreted into the small intestine, is highly alkaline.

For the pH level of bile and selected other body fluids, see Table 7.2.

If the concentration of positively charged hydrogen ions in any of the body fluids increases, it causes the pH measurement of that fluid to move toward 0. This is referred to as an "acid shift." On the other hand, if the concentration of negatively charged hydroxyl ions in any of the body fluids increases, it causes the pH measurement of that fluid to move toward 14. This is referred to as an "alkaline shift."

Mechanisms That Control the pH of Body Fluids

The body uses several mechanisms to control the pH levels of its fluids. For example, lactic acid, which is produced during normal muscular activity, is a weak acid. It does not dissociate much—that is, it loses relatively few hydrogen ions to the blood—but like any acid, if it isn't

Table 7.2. The pH of Body Fluids		
Fluid	**Typical pH Range**	**Characteristics**
Gastric secretions	1.0–3.5	Most acidic substance in the body
Urine	4.5–8.0	Can fall within wide range, depending on wastes
Saliva	6.0–7.0	Nearly neutral
Venous blood	7.3–7.35	Very close to neutral, but slightly alkaline; tightly controlled
Arterial blood	7.45	Very close to neutral, but slightly alkaline; tightly controlled
Small intestine secretions	7.5–8.0	Slightly alkaline
Bile	7.8–8.2	Most alkaline substance in the body

buffered, it will lose enough that acidity will gradually build up, leading to acidosis. Baking soda, produced in large quantities naturally in the body, buffers (neutralizes) lactic acid, rendering it less harmful. It converts lactic acid to carbonic acid, a weaker and less damaging acid than lactic acid. The amount of carbonic acid in the blood goes up slightly because the excess lactic acid is converted to carbonic acid. The amount of bicarbonate (mainly in the form of sodium bicarbonate) in the blood goes down slightly because the neutralizing bicarbonate becomes part of the newly formed carbonic acid. The hydrogen concentration in the blood increases slightly, but by less than what is caused by lactic acid.

Buffering mechanisms cannot completely prevent blood hydrogen concentration from increasing. The system just minimizes the damaging increase. The net effect is that the blood pH decreases slightly—that is, it becomes more acid.

The body is so geared toward reducing accumulating acid pH that it will sacrifice almost anything in the effort. It will even cannibalize its own skeleton, the mineral bank that contains a lifetime savings account of alkaline minerals, to neutralize temporarily damaging acids.

Buffer Systems

The pH must remain within a very narrow range for the metabolism to function properly. If the pH of any tissue falls outside the proper band, cellular function will lessen or the body will die. So it is obviously critical that the body regulate the pH of all of these various fluids in order to survive, or at least to function effectively. To safeguard our lives, the body has created several elaborate systems that carefully monitor pH. If any aberrant acid-alkaline deviations take place, it will quickly control the situation to restore the balance, if possible. These regulation and control systems, designed to correct these fluctuations, are the acid-base buffer systems.

If we were to take in any strong acids (unlikely, as they aren't found in normal foods), those compounds would almost immediately dissociate into large quantities of hydrogen and hydroxyl ions, creating drastic changes in the blood pH.

A buffer is defined as a solution containing two or more chemical compounds that prevent major alterations in pH, regardless of whether an acid or a base was to be added to the solution.

The body's three buffer systems that are the most metabolically active and therefore the most significant are:

1. The bicarbonate–carbon dioxide system—bicarbonate buffers acids, resulting in carbonic acid being formed from water and carbon dioxide.
2. The extracellular system—made up mainly of the proportional concentration of phosphate.
3. The skeletal bone system—bones continuously release their alkaline minerals, including magnesium, manganese, sodium, potassium, zinc, boron, copper, strontium, and calcium.

Much of the carbonic acid that ends up in the blood from the buffering process finds its way into the red blood cells, where it becomes buffered by the potassium salt of hemoglobin. This is another reason to keep your potassium intake high!

The largest alkaline reservoir in the body is in the pancreas. This organ produces high concentrations of bicarbonate in the digestive fluid it dumps into the small intestine.

The bile produced in the liver and stored in the gallbladder is also highly alkaline. Bile also dumps into the small intestine. Ayurveda considers the bile to be the most intense (pitta) fluid in the body.

Stomach acid is the body's acid reservoir. The majority of hydrogen ions are right there in that superacidic stomach juice.

Acids are produced by the body during the normal process of cell function. Their production is increased greatly during stress and sympathetic nervous system stimulation. The rate and concentration of the body's metabolic acids increases with exercise. The largest culprit in excess acid production is the cellular oxidation of fats, carbohydrates, and proteins, the very macronutrients that nourish us and keep us alive.

The intricate network of powerful buffers is very complex and very efficient, so that variations in the pH of the major bodily fluids do not often occur. The body is bombarded by acids on a moment-by-moment basis—just by being alive! Internal metabolic processes and sources from outside all contribute to this stress. It is this unending onslaught of acids that begins to drain the efficiency of the organic buffers, as well as exhaust the neutralizing chemicals (especially cell and bone minerals) that facilitate proper buffer functioning.

In a healthy person, the daily oxidation of foods produces a wide array of chemical components that acutely impact the acid-base condition. The cellular oxidation of carbohydrates and fats produces a disproportionate quantity of carbon dioxide, which finds its way into venous blood. This carbon dioxide is ultimately toxic if it is not processed, and stressful to the body and metabolism as a whole.

A trace amount of carbon dioxide will be vented out through the lungs, depending on the efficiency of the respiratory system. But the entire body has to remove more than 30 liters of carbonic acid daily. This is an astonishing amount of acid. So well buffered are these acid wastes that arterial blood and venous blood have almost identical amounts of hydrogen ions.

The remaining concentration of this toxic carbon dioxide, the amount that does not exit the lungs, will combine with water to produce carbonic acid, shifting the pH of the blood to the acid side. This carbonic acid then needs to be buffered by alkaline buffering compounds in the body, including calcium and other alkaline minerals from bone. Any excess remaining unbuffered is eliminated through the kidneys.

Respiratory and Urinary Mechanisms of pH Control

Respiration through the lungs is critical for pH balance. Every time you breath out, water and carbon dioxide exit the body in the exhaled breath. The carbon dioxide comes from the venous blood moving through the capillaries of the lungs. Therefore, the returning oxygenated arterial blood contains less carbonic acid and a slightly higher (more alkaline) pH. Remember how important deep, full breathing is to keeping pH in tight balance.

If you hold your breath or breathe shallowly, the carbon dioxide in the blood is increased. Carbonic acid has to form, and the blood pH heads farther toward acid. Anything that reduces respiration or lung-gas exchange can produce acidosis, sometimes quite dramatically.

The kidneys are big players in controlling blood pH. They are capable of eliminating much larger amounts of acid than the lungs. In a pinch, they can also excrete base, which the lungs cannot. This makes the kidneys the last emergency control mechanism for pH problems. The kidneys reclaim the tremendous amount of bicarbonate that the body needs to balance cell acids. This process requires sodium, so that valuable mineral ends up being lost in the urine and has to be consumed regularly.

The pH of the various fluids in the body varies from an extremely acid 1.0 in the stomach to a mildly alkaline 8.2 in the bile. Yet the blood is so tightly controlled that we will never see variation there in even the sickest patient. Modern medicine is very focused on blood tests, yet that procedure is unlikely to reveal any significant information about pH. In fact, standard blood tests don't routinely include a test for pH.

The body is extremely efficient at buffering the acid load produced by normal living. It neutralizes these huge quantities with little difficulty. But if the buffer systems fall behind, the body will not hesitate to sacrifice its own skeleton to provide the alkaline minerals needed to keep the pH in the proper range. Therefore, it's critical to have a way to assess body chemistry, through symptoms or chemistry, and a scheme to monitor changes.

We can gain a lot of insight into body balancing from studying the scientific perspective. Scientists have learned a lot about pH and its critical importance in metabolic functioning. Even so, this information has not made much headway in modern medicine. While conventional medicine recognizes cases of extreme pH crisis, such as respiratory acidosis, very little investigation has been done in the scientific mainstream into the importance of using pH as a predictor of health or of the importance of keeping pH in tight control with diet and natural medicine. But according to the experts in this field, this is the next new frontier in health awareness in the United States.

8

The Modern Understanding of Body Balance in Alternative Medicine

Conventional medicine might not be quick to recognize and implement these *Body Balance* ideas, but a growing number of alternative physicians and researchers are coming to the conclusion that pH balance is critical to regaining and maintaining lifelong health. Increasingly, evidence is accumulating that supports the importance of controlling acid load.

We are now finding out that just about everything we do generates excess acid that must be buffered, at the expense of our skeleton and mood. Eating most foods creates acids. Having infections or allergies does too, as does having stress. It turns out that many of the practices recommended by leading naturopathic physicians and holistic medical doctors are right on the money, and we might just be getting some verification for why these methods work: They balance pH.

Alternative medicine proponents advocate eating a whole foods diet. Fruits and vegetables, in particular, are at the forefront of everyone's dietary suggestions. It turns out that they also help to keep pH in balance. Whole grains? They are absorbed more slowly, so they require less buffering to control the spike in blood acid. They also contain valuable alkaline buffering minerals. Scientific studies are now emerging that confirm the benefit of such a diet, one that effectively keeps pH in balance, for muscle, bone, and joint health. Ditto for cardiovascular disease, lung conditions, kidney diseases, bacterial infection, and menopause.

Alternative and complementary practitioners have always maintained that "hot" emotions, like anger, are destructive to good health. Now we know that reactive emotions and stress provoke acidity, while more passive behavior creates an alkaline pH. Alternative researchers working with pH have shown that a program designed to balance pH over one year successfully treated some very mentally sick people.

Of course, sugar is the ultimate no-no in natural healing. Sugar increases acid load. Scientists have found that limiting sugar and refined grains brings about big reductions in antisocial behavior, suicides, and violence. So it seems that the natural healing advocates have been right all along—and we can expect the news to spread and have a big impact in the health world.

The Experts Concur

Susan E. Brown, Ph.D., C.C.N., of East Syracuse, New York, is a medical anthropologist and certified nutritionist. She holds a doctorate degree from the University of Michigan and is the recipient of two Fulbright-Hays Scholar Awards, has an Organization of American States Research Fellowship, and is a member of Sigma Xi, the honorary scientific research organization of North America.

Dr. Brown consults extensively on socioeconomic, cultural, educational, and health issues. She has taught in North and South American universities and has authored numerous articles published in academic journals and popular magazines. Currently, Dr. Brown directs the Osteoporosis Education Project and the Nutrition Education and Consulting Service in East Syracuse, where she conducts primary research and lectures on osteoporosis prevention and reversal. She also teaches the Better Bones, Better Body Program, a holistic, natural program for rejuvenating bone health, and serves as a consultant to numerous medical groups, including Serammune Physicians Laboratory in Sterling, Virginia.

According to Dr. Brown, humans evolved in the ocean, an alkaline environment. And our body's internal environment is still alkaline today, with a pH just above 7.0. Our enzymes, immune system, and repair mechanisms all work best at an alkaline pH.

Overall, Dr. Brown says, we want our internal balance to be slightly alkaline to function optimally. But our biochemical functioning, the metabolism of food, and frankly, just the processes of living in a human body produce a lot of acid by-products. When we exercise, we produce lactic acid and carbon dioxide. As we saw in Chapter 7, lactic acid, with a pH of under 7.0, adds to the total acid load of the body. In the process of respiration and metabolism, carbon dioxide turns into carbonic acid in the water of the body's fluids.

Eating food also creates acids. For example, when we consume the sulfur and phosphorus contained in meats, grains, and beans, we generate sulfuric acid and phosphoric acid. Dr. Brown goes on to say that immune responses, such as allergies, hypersensitivities, and even stress, generate substantial amounts of acidic products. To regain what she calls "the life-supporting alkaline state," the body must buffer these acids, from whatever original source, by combining them with alkaline minerals. Dr. Brown points out that acid-forming elements in our food include phosphorus, sulfur, chlorine, and iodine. When these elements predominate in a food and the food is metabolized, it leaves an acid state. Minerals that produce an alkaline state when metabolized include calcium, magnesium, potassium, sodium, chromium, selenium, and iron.

To maintain life, the body requires innumerable chemical reactions to take place. These reactions can only occur within a very specific pH range. As we discussed earlier, the body has many checks and balances to preserve pH within a tight range. Most of these balancing mechanisms require alkaline minerals to buffer accumulated acids. When you eat a surplus of acid-forming minerals and a shortfall of alkalinizing minerals, body buffering mineral pools can be depleted. The intracellular fluid becomes acidotic.

According to Dr. Brown, an underlying metabolic acidity is a shared trait among, and a probable causative feature to, all degenerative and autoimmune diseases. An acid condition stresses cell metabolism in several ways. It impairs energy production, encourages fluid retention and edema, and typically increases free radical production. It is essential to reestablish the health-promoting alkaline state to renew proper immune function and overall health.

When lymphocytes eat up foreign particles, they produce acid. So, when your immune system is stressed by accumulations of undesirable waste materials, the very act of cleaning up makes you even more acid.

Maintaining proper pH is a critical function for the body. Many organs participate. The kidneys, adrenals, and lungs all play important roles. Tom Drost, M.D., is a general surgeon with holistic leanings who practices in Seattle, Washington. An instructor in general surgery at Bastyr University, Dr. Drost recently graduated with an additional doctorate in naturopathic medicine. Dr. Drost uses pH status for diagnosis of some possible underlying chronic health concerns. He maintains that acid blood pH can be a sign of excess lactic acid in the body. "This can be a sign of exercise beyond capacity, damaged muscle tissue, or lack of circulation to outlying tissues," he says. "Alkalinizing measures are used to balance the excess lactic acid in the tissues. The underlying tissue problems must be treated appropriately."

Even more important, declares Dr. Brown, is diet. If you eat a balanced, whole foods diet, the net acid-alkaline balance is upheld in proper proportion. A diet high in animal protein, sugar, caffeine, and processed foods can cause the body's pH to drift toward the acid side. And that's exactly the diet we mainly consume in our culture. As our diet pushes us toward an acid state, our body responds by withdrawing alkalinizing minerals, especially calcium, from the blood and the storehouses in the tissues. The majority of fruits and vegetables leave an alkalizing effect. Most grains and high-protein foods are somewhat acid generating.

According to Dr. Susan Lark, all this wear and tear of daily life gradually adds up to cause our cells to lose their healthy alkalinity and become more acidic. We become more susceptible to disease. She claims that more than 90 percent of Americans become overly acidic during their lifetimes (and presumably continue that way unless they take measures to reverse the trend). Dr. Lark concurs that this is mainly due to diet. One hallmark of being generally overacid, she says, is taking over-the-counter remedies for stomach upset or chronic allergies.

Dr. Robin Dipasquale calls this the "cooking ground for chronic disease." Dr. Theodore Baroody, a bit more radical, suggests that virtually all symptoms to which humans fall prey are the result of this fundamental pH imbalance. He describes a cascade of symptoms that escalate through stages as the pH slips consistently and the body becomes more acidotic. As you can imagine, it's a long list.

Dr. Baroody's beginning symptoms include acne, muscle pain, cold hands and feet, hyperactivity, constipation, and irregular heartbeat. As the condition progresses, he includes the intermediate symptoms of cold sores, depression, memory loss, migraine, asthma, hives, impotence, and colitis. Advanced symptoms include an array of all the chronic degenerative diseases: Crohn's disease, lupus, rheumatoid arthritis, and scleroderma.

Problem Areas

To sum up, there is a predictable set of factors that promote acid metabolism. Stress tops the list. Strenuous exercise, especially in an untrained body and combined with improper diet and lifestyle habits, also ups the body's acid burden. The diet can be a big contributor. Animal protein, including milk products, refined sugar and flour, caffeine, cola drinks (containing phosphoric acid), and alcohol are all risk factors.

Certain drugs can be a problem, so it's good to check with your practitioner. Being in midlife ups acidity. Remember, pitta, the inflammatory dosha, dominates from age twenty to age sixty. Food allergies, especially to milk products, wheat, peanuts, corn, and soybeans, can contribute. In particular, allergies to the amines contained in tomatoes, oranges, wine, chocolate, and Parmesan cheese are problematic.

So how will you know that your pH is off? Remember that most, but not all, Americans have an overall pH that is too low—on the acid side. Acidotic people often experience fatigue, even after enough hours of sleep. They have joint aches and pains and frequent heartburn, which is also called gastritis or gastroesophageal reflux (GERD). They may get sick a lot with colds and flu or have chronic urinary infections or chronic allergies or chemical sensitivities. Sometimes, a glass of wine with dinner makes their nose run. They have acne, irritability, dizziness, depression, memory loss, and insomnia.

People with acid bodies often have chronic inflammatory conditions, such as "hot" asthma, bursitis, tendonitis, colitis, or PMS. To top it off, they may suffer low libido, diarrhea, malodorous urine, headache, and rapid breathing.

Rarely, people go to the alkaline side. Even though this is uncommon, it is no healthier. Balance is the goal. Overly alkaline folks have symptoms of chronic low body temperature, chronic excess mucus, "wet" asthma, muscle soreness, cramps, bone spurs, edema (especially in the hands), hyperventilation, numbness, prickling sensations, and "full"-type indigestion that is successfully decreased by supplementing with hydrochloric acid.

Mental Functions, Mood, and Behavior

Your body pH can affect your mood, outlook on life, and day-to-day energy. Dr. Dipasquale also holds that the emotions you experience can affect the ultimate pH of your body. "Hot" emotions, like easy anger (pitta), provoke more acidity, while more passive behavior (kapha) brings on more alkalinity.

Dr. Brown looks at acid behavior as stress, which results in cortisol secretion, which in turn adds to the acid load, prompting a person to aggressive behavior. Alkaline behavior, by comparison, is more passive and calm.

Dr. Lark brings up one example of how your acid-alkaline imbalance can affect you. She says that overacidity depresses the central nervous system, causing feelings of depression. An acid pH can cause us to lose our desire to be "social," she says. It directly affects our ability to cope with life and to stay positive. We may become introverted, ill-tempered, and intolerant.

Fortunately, alkalinity acts as a mood elevator.

People with work involving intense mental activity and concentration create large amounts of acid. The body's ability to buffer acids can have a hard time keeping up with the brain drain.

Scientific research has shown that the brain demands a lot of energy. It makes up only 2 percent of the body's weight, but it consumes more than 20 percent of the body's energy. Scientists think that the brain is incapable of storing significant amounts of blood sugar. It requires a constant supply through the blood. As mental activity increases, so too does the brain's requirement for energy in the form of oxygen and glucose.[1]

Putting on your thinking cap causes your brain to burn oxygen at a higher rate, cutting into your alkaline reserves. If you, like many people, breathe with shallow breaths when pounding away on the computer, you inhale less oxygen. More acidic carbon dioxide is then retained. The lack of movement and circulation, allowing wastes to build up in the tissues, doesn't help. Keeping alkaline reserves high, breathing with deep cleansing breaths, and taking a break for a few minutes every hour or so can help you stay sharp.

In a placebo-controlled study published in 1987, 296 subjects were selected because they suffered from various psychological disturbances. These were sick people; they suffered from autism, dementia, schizophrenia, bipolar disorder, anxiety, and a grab bag of other mental illnesses.

The scientists measured the patients' venous blood pH in a controlled way over an eight-hour time span, after the subjects had eaten a series of predefined meals. Each subject was placed on a pH-balancing dietary supplement program, individualized according to the subject's pH measurements, for one year.

The researchers performed psychological tests (the Minnesota Multiphasic Personality Inventory) before the study began, and the patients kept a wellness-index diary to monitor symptoms on a daily basis. About 86 percent of the individuals experienced substantial reduction or complete elimination of their symptoms within the year. Many patients improved to the extent that psychotherapy was no longer necessary. Of these, 84 percent reached that milestone within 120 days of starting the pH-balancing program.[2] Although the scientists were not specifically studying physical illnesses, physicians monitoring the patients reported that many had substantial improvement in a host of physical conditions (including pancreatitis, cystitis, fibrocystic breast, dysmenorrhea, and skin infections). Are we surprised?

Another double-blind study looked at the effects of reducing the consumption of acid-producing, refined, sugary foods on 3,000 incarcerated juvenile delinquents. Eliminating these triggers brought about a 21 percent reduction in antisocial behavior, a 100 percent reduction in suicides, a 25 percent reduction in assaults, and a 75 percent reduction in the use of restraints, when compared with study controls.[3]

Dr. Brown recommends a diet composed of about 35 percent acid-forming foods and 65 percent alkaline-forming foods. To accomplish this, eat two servings of alkaline foods for every one serving of acid foods. Dr. Baroody goes even farther with his eighty-twenty rule. He maintains that 99.85 percent of people on the planet should consume 80 percent (eight of ten servings) of alkaline-forming foods and only 20 percent (two of ten servings) of acid-forming foods.[4]

Adjusting pH with Supplements

Often, dietary adjustment for pH can be a slow process for people who are far over the line. Nutritional supplements may help to speed the journey to pH balance. Nutrients that produce alkalis include the minerals calcium, magnesium, potassium, sodium, chromium, selenium, iron, zinc, manganese, boron, copper, strontium, and several miscellaneous trace minerals. Other dietary supplements to consider include algae (spirulina or chlorella), barley grass or wheat grass, bee pollen, royal jelly, nutritional yeast, chlorophyll, pepsin, digestive enzymes, beta-carotene, and vitamin B-complex. Alkaline-producing foods include vegetables and fruits in general and perhaps sea salt.

On the off chance that you need to acidify your overall pH, minerals that produce acids include phosphorus, sulfur, chlorine, and iodine. Foods that acidify include refined sugar (although it's not a good food to consume for other reasons); protein from egg, beef, pork, and chicken; and cheese.

Body Balance and Healthy Bones

Proper pH balance is particularly important in sustaining correct mineral status and, consequently, bone health.

Calcium composes 1 to 2 percent of adult human body weight. More than 99 percent of an adult body's entire calcium content is found in the teeth and bones.[5]

Dr. Brown maintains that the countries that have the lowest calcium levels in the diet—such as Peru, Sri Lanka, and China—have populations that maintain lifelong healthy bones, while Americans have brittle bones. This, she says, is because Western populations have overburdened themselves with an excessive acid load, throwing pH out of balance.

"The most important of all bone-affecting balances, however, is the least well known," says Dr. Brown. "This equilibrium involves the delicate chemical balance of acid and alkaline within our bodies." Internal acids damage our internal environment just like acid rain causes havoc with the environment outside. Without even realizing it, most of us devour diets high in acid-forming foods.

This results in chronic, low-grade acidosis. Modern clinicians, including Dr. Brown, are beginning to look at chronic metabolic acidosis as the key unseen cause of osteoporosis. It seems that just a slight lean toward the acid side generates osteoporosis. The body then has to take valuable alkaline salts of bone-building minerals (magnesium, manganese, sodium, potassium, zinc, boron, copper, strontium, and calcium) from bone tissue and use them to buffer those internal acids. Your skeleton, in addition to holding you up, is the vast reserve storehouse for these minerals, so they are withdrawn to fit the need. Nature never thought we would need to make continual withdrawals from this storage depot. But now we are. Acidosis *is* a mineral deficiency, especially a deficiency of valuable potassium.[6]

William Lee Cowden, M.D., practices integrated medicine at the Conservative Medicine Institute in Richardson, Texas. Dr. Cowden says that acid-neutralizing calcium comes first from blood and soft tissue. He says that this initial depletion of muscle calcium can cause muscle cramps. When calcium begins to be pulled from bone, it can end up being deposited as calcium salts in joints, eventually causing degenerative arthritis.[7]

Researchers at the Osteoporosis Education Project have realized that internal acid load is a major factor behind the osteoporosis epidemic. To counteract this, they encourage a diet high in alkalinizing foods, such as fruits, vegetables, nuts, spices, herbs, seasonings, seeds, and pulses, including lentils. They have found that people in other cultures who eat closer to this type of diet do better with less calcium because less mineral is wasted for buffering.[8]

Roberta Lee, M.D., is the medical director of the Center for Health and Healing at Beth Israel Medical Center in New York City. She practices complementary medicine with a specialty in herbal therapeutics. Dr. Lee sees a lot of osteoporosis at her clinic. She reminds us that hypochlorhydria is common in aging people. To check out the possibility of urinary calcium loss, she suggests testing for the level of urinary N-teleopeptides (NTx). Measuring the day's second urine, NTx is an assessment of the urinary excretion of calcium, according to Dr. Lee. "If NTx is out of the normal range," says Dr. Lee, "it might indicate calcium loss from bone, and a person might be at risk. It is an inference of osteoporosis," she claims.[9]

Dr. Lee uses calcium citrate, a source of calcium bonded to the weak citric acid, or calcium hydroxyapatite, the form in which calcium is stored in the bones. Hydroxyapatite calcium has consistently been shown to be the form that most effectively prevents or reverses bone loss. Since the hydroxyapatite form is possibly of animal bone origin, she cautions us to make sure the product has been evaluated for lead content.

Robert J. Peshek, D.D.S., was a pioneering nutritional dentist writing in the 1970s. He wrote *Balancing Body Chemistry with Nutrition*, a book that was way ahead of its time. Dr. Peshek greatly praised calcium lactate, another very absorbable form.

Lynne August, M.D., received her medical degree from Washington

University School of Medicine in 1973. She is the founder and director of Health Equations, a service that offers health professionals and patients an innovative, objective evaluation of a standard blood test. Dr. August was a clinical researcher at the Institute of Applied Biology in New York, where she participated in research on nontoxic therapeutic lipids. She also draws upon her training and practice in Ayurveda.

The Health Equations evaluation tells patients which metabolic track they are on and where it will lead, even decades from now. Based on thirty years of clinical medical research, the Health Equations Blood Test Evaluation provides a snapshot of a person's nutritional status with concise, personalized interpretations and recommendations. Follow-up evaluations examine a person's response to the recommendations.

Dr. August has an excellent system of classifying nutrients and body processes into two categories: anabolic and catabolic. This perspective is valuable in helping us get a handle on where to start with classifying foods and minerals.

According to Dr. August, many individuals are calcium deficient because their bodies do not absorb the calcium from the foods they eat. She says patients lose calcium for a number of reasons:

- When tissue and cell cholesterol is high, calcium is lost in their urine
- When tissue and cell cholesterol is low, calcium is bound up and not available to the cells
- When processed foods are consumed, calcium is used for buffering
- When insufficient protein and/or fat is eaten or digested, calcium cannot be stored in the skeleton
- When the diet is inadequate, insufficient calcium is consumed.[10]

In Chapter 9, we will examine a scheme for measuring your average pH levels over several days. Based on your calculations, you can adjust the type of calcium you use therapeutically according to your average pH status. Remember, vitamin C will acidify and vitamin D will alkalinize. If your pH is below 6.0 (too acid), add alkaline calcium carbonate. If your pH is in the 5.6 to 6.0 range, add 1,000 to 2,000 international units of vitamin D once or twice a day to help normalize the chemistry. Do not take vitamin C. If your pH dips as low as from 5.2 to 5.6, some experts suggest taking amounts of up to 5,000 international units of vitamin D. Below 5.0, some experts use up to 10,000 international units of vitamin

D a day, since little vitamin D is absorbed in the acid environment. When you reach the ideal pH range of 6.0 to 7.0, cut back on the calcium carbonate and vitamin D, and go to a more neutral calcium form.

If your average pH is between 6.0 and 7.0 (the ideal range), just use the neutral calcium forms (gluconate and orotate). These will support your total reserve of alkalinity, but will not move your pH precipitously. Use these neutral forms of calcium in concert with an array of nutritive trace minerals.

If your pH is above 7.0 (too alkaline), do not take vitamin D, and utilize calcium lactate (formed with the mild acid, lactic acid) and vitamin C (a mild acid). A dose of about 1,000 milligrams twice a day of vitamin C is likely to work well. The higher above pH 7.0 you are, the more vitamin C you can tolerate. As you begin to acidify and your pH number goes down, switch from the lactate form to a less acidic form of calcium.

Dr. Brown considers chronic low-grade metabolic acidosis to be a major, and generally overlooked, factor contributing to the development of osteoporosis among Westernized populations. For most individuals, the role that metabolic acidosis plays in the development of osteoporosis is as important as, if not more important than, that played by hormonal balance. Magnesium and potassium levels go down even before the calcium level does. Dr. Brown promotes an alkalinizing program that includes foods and supplements. She calls this new mineral-rich diet the Alkaline Way. She says that eating this Alkaline Way diet moves people from metabolic acidity toward a life-supporting alkaline chemistry. Her book, *Better Bones, Better Body* (Contemporary Books, 2000), goes into greater detail on the Alkaline Way Diet.

Scientists in the Nephrology Unit of the University of Rochester School of Medicine and Dentistry in New York confirm that modern humans tend to consume a diet that generates metabolic acids, leading to a reduction in the concentration of systemic bicarbonate and a fall in pH. Metabolic acidosis causes a release of calcium from bone that initially is simply due to the mineral actually dissolving. On a more chronic basis, metabolic acidosis alters bone cell function, they say. There is an increase in bone resorption caused by osteoclasts and a decrease in bone formation by osteoblasts. Because kidney function declines as we age, we are less able to excrete these metabolic acids. According to the scientists, a slight but significant metabolic acidosis leads to greater loss of bone mineral and an increased potential to fracture.[11]

Studies show that feeding animals sulfur-containing amino acids such as cysteine and methionine, which are abundant in animal protein, causes a reduction in bone density.[12] Rats fed a diet of 15 percent soy protein as a control did not have this bone loss. Researchers theorize that homocysteine reacts with collagen in the body's connective tissues, hastening bone breakdown.

Beans, peas, and other legumes, including lentils, are excellent sources of protein. If you include these in your diet and also eat whole grains such as whole wheat, oats, corn, barley, millet, buckwheat, and rice, these two food groups together will provide the entire assortment of essential amino acids you need for protein. Legumes are high in the alkaline minerals calcium, magnesium, potassium, iron, copper, zinc, and vitamin B-complex, all nutrients that benefit strong bones. As an added benefit, legumes are high in soluble fiber, the kind that lowers cholesterol.

This said, remember that it's still necessary to consume enough protein. Dr. August cites several studies correlating dietary protein and bone density. Femur (thigh bone) density is associated with the amount of protein in the diet. The femur is composed of a very important protein matrix in which minerals are deposited. Unless there is sufficient dietary protein, the body cannot preserve this protein matrix. So, as with most things, balance is the key: We need neither too much nor too little protein.

The Framingham Osteoporosis Study, published in 2002, measured bone mineral density in 907 subjects. The scientists also concluded that a diet high in fruit and vegetable intake appears to be protective in men. In fact, the men who ate the most fruits and vegetables had the best bone mass in the study, regardless of other dietary factors.[13]

You will notice that a fruit and vegetable diet, while dramatically beneficial, has not been a focus of recent media attention or public awareness, which has gone instead toward the importance of calcium. While calcium is no doubt important, especially in a culture that eats a high-acid diet, we need to take a holistic approach toward the total diet. Clearly, something as simple as getting the nationally recommended five servings of vegetables and fruits (which almost no American actually does) may be equally as important as consuming adequate calcium when it comes to preserving bone density.

And some vegetables, particularly carrots, do contain considerable calcium. Leafy green vegetables pack a substantial dose of calcium, as well as iron and magnesium.

Dr. Lark likes fruits for their potassium content. This alkalinizing mineral—found in bananas, oranges, berries, peaches, apricots, and melons—offsets the drain on the alkaline minerals in your bones and decreases fluid retention.

Body Balance and Cardiovascular Disease

Women: Eat your fruit and veggies. Your heart will thank you for it. At least, that's the indication of a new study in a recent issue of *The American Journal of Clinical Nutrition*. Women who ate between four and ten servings of fruits and vegetables per day reduced their risk of cardiovascular disease by between 20 percent and 30 percent.[14] Women without any cardiovascular risk factors, such as diabetes or hypertension, fared even better. This news shouldn't surprise you. The researchers said that the 20 to 30 percent reduction in risk associated with increased intake of fruits and vegetables might be a conservative estimate, owing to measurement techniques.

The data came from almost 40,000 women health professionals, all with no known history of cardiovascular disease, who took part in the Women's Health Study. They recorded total servings of twenty-eight vegetables and sixteen fruits eaten per day and were monitored for an average of five years for incidence of heart attack, stroke, coronary angioplasty, coronary bypass, and death due to cardiovascular disease.

The scientists maintain that it's probably part of this whole picture we've been seeing concerning plant foods and the health benefits for heart disease. It's probable that, in addition to the antioxidants, vitamins, minerals, and plant hormones found in food plants, other enzymes and hormones, which both protect the plant from fungus or help to pollinate it, may help prevent disease in humans. You will notice that the findings are right in line with what Dr. Brown and other experts are suggesting. (For another reason to eat a diet high in plant foods, see below.)

Homocysteine

Here's another reason to stay away from acid-forming high-protein diets. One of the amino acids that is abundant in animal protein is the sulfur-containing compound methionine. Homocysteine, a toxic waste product, is generated form the breakdown of methionine. It is now clear that homocysteine damages the vascular endothelial cells, contributing to blood clots and heart attacks.[15] Homocysteine levels are a good predictor of heart disease risk.

Recent advances in the understanding of homocysteine chemistry begin to explain the action of this toxic substance. Apparently, homocysteine reacts with proteins in the body's connective tissues, causing them to break down permanently. This leads to a collection of related connective tissue disorders, in addition to the venous connective tissue damage. These diseases, common in later life, include cognitive decline, presbyopia (age-related farsightedness), and of course, osteoporosis.[16]

A recent study found that vegetarians have high blood levels of salicylic acid, the anti-inflammatory ingredient in aspirin. Scientists suggest that this may partly explain why people who eat a diet rich in fruits and vegetables generally have a lower incidence of heart disease and cancer.[17] Cinnamon has one of the highest concentrations of salicylic acid.

So, it looks as if one of the most profound things a healthcare professional can do is to encourage clients to eat a healthy diet—and for almost everybody, that means more alkaline.

Body Balance and Menopause

It is widely understood that women after menopause have a greater risk of calcium depletion and resultant osteoporosis. It looks pretty likely that postmenopausal women can stop the progress of bone loss by getting their net acid down.

Measuring how much calcium is being excreted through the kidney is one way to evaluate the loss of minerals that would be better staying in bone. The chronic low-grade metabolic acidosis that occurs in normal people from dietary net acid load and age-related kidney functional decline may contribute to osteoporosis by increasing urine calcium excretion.

To back up Dr. Brown's assertion, a study in the journal *Kidney International* showed that administering potassium bicarbonate, a strong alkaline mineral, substantially reduced the urinary excretion of calcium associated with osteoporosis.[18] The research was done by a leading kidney researcher with a specialty in acid load, Lynda Frassetto, M.D., assistant clinical professor of medicine at the University of California, San Francisco. Of course, potassium is a strong chemical that should be used only under a doctor's supervision. Dr. Brown says that comparable changes can be gained in menopause with an alkaline diet emphasizing vegetables, fruits, and nuts.[19]

The vagina is supposed to have an acidic pH (between 4.0 and 5.0). This prevents harmful fungi and bacteria from flourishing there. In menopause, the estrogen deficiency changes the vagina to an alkaline pH. Monitor overall body pH and adjust as necessary to keep the menopausal vagina acidic. Test the vagina secretions directly with pH paper. If they're not in the 4.0 to 5.0 range, something needs to be done. Generally, adjusting the overall diet and lifestyle to correct the pH of other tissues will nudge the vagina to its proper pH. Vagina pH drift is caused by estrogen deficiency, so if the general pH procedures outlined in this book do not restore postmenopausal vaginal pH, it's time for a specialist.

Body Balance and the Lungs

The lungs are critical for maintaining proper acidity in the body. Recall that carbon dioxide can exit the lungs, reducing the amount that would be available to combine with water to create carbonic acid. The net effect is to lower total acid in the body. In high-acid conditions, the lungs receive a message to work harder to expel the excess carbon dioxide. Eventually, the lungs become stressed and damaged.

When a buildup of blood carbon dioxide produces a shift in the body's pH balance and causes the system to become more acidic, it's called respiratory acidosis, and it can be a result of a problem either involving the respiratory system or signals from the brain that control breathing.[20] The blood pH will be below 7.35. The main symptom is difficult breathing, possibly followed by headache, drowsiness, restlessness, tremor, and confusion. Sometimes, the body responds with mechanisms of metabolic alkalosis, which may produce cyanosis, a bluish skin discoloration. Severe cases lead to coma and death.

Dr. Cowden reminds us that oxygen will bind to hemoglobin of red blood cells only within a very limited range of pH in the lung. If lung pH is tilted, airway microbes can grow much more easily, resulting in respiratory infection such as cold or bronchitis.

Dr. Drost points out that patients with severe lung disease, such as chronic obstructive pulmonary disease (COPD), tend to retain carbon dioxide. This causes them to feel as if they are chronically not getting enough air. Under these conditions, the brain "resets" the pH feedback mechanism and normalizes the breathing, reducing the carbon dioxide associated "drive" to breathe, and leaving the carbon dioxide level permanently high. We know from our discussion that high carbon dioxide promotes high acidity, kidney stress, and bone loss. He suggests that this pH balance problem can be balanced with food and supplements.[21] Dr. Drost uses naturopathic therapies (diet, minerals, and herbs) to restore balance.

In normal fat metabolism, acid compounds called ketones are routinely produced and find their way to the bloodstream. One way the body attempts to balance the pH is to cause hard breathing to eliminate the acid-producing pH. People who cannot metabolize fats but eat high-fat diets may be at risk for acidosis and respiratory stress.

Even though only a small amount of carbon dioxide is expelled through the breath, it is still important. Deep, full breaths are healthy!

Body Balance and the Kidneys

The body is composed mostly of water. This water—in the fluids outside of the cells—contains salt in the same proportion found in the ocean. The chemistry of this salt is the primary mechanism for moving water around in the body.

Dr. Drost says that patients with chronic renal disease and other similar metabolic disorders have chronic pH derangements.

According to Dr. August, lack of thirst is a positive sign that you are dehydrated. If your internal chemistry is out of balance, your tastes can't be trusted. If you are not normally thirsty, Dr. August suggests that you start by eating salt until you begin to have a taste for it. Then start drinking water—habitually at first. Over months, or even over years, you will eventually develop a normal thirst.

I have definitely seen this to be true in practice. The body accommodates to the normal water consumption by regulating kidney function. People who get used to drinking less water (to reduce bathroom trips, for example) stop getting thirsty. They can't trust their own desire to drink and end up with concentrated waste in the urine.

Once your tastes are normalized, Dr. August says to drink water according to your thirst and eat salt according to your taste. Remember, caffeinated and alcoholic beverages cause loss of water from the tissues.

Dr. Cowden mentions that the calcium the body sacrifices to buffer acids in the blood eventually ends up in the urine. If that mineral excess ends up collecting in the small tubules of the kidney or bladder, you will be at risk for urinary stones. It is best to keep the calcium in the bank—in the bone—in the first place.

There are certain kidney and endocrine diseases in which water or salt restriction is absolutely vital. Some people with high blood pressure need to watch their salt intake. Those people should monitor their condition medically.

Bacterial Dysbiosis

Leo Galland, M.D., is a researcher who has focused his studies on dysbiosis, a state of disordered microbial ecology that causes disease. The dysbiosis concept rests on the assumption that patterns of intestinal flora, specifically overgrowth of certain common intestinal microorganisms, have an impact on human health.[22] Dysbiosis is thought to contribute to chronic intestinal disorders including irritable bowel disease, inflammatory or autoimmune disorders, food allergy, atopic eczema, unexplained fatigue, arthritis and ankylosing spondylitis, malnutrition, neuropsychiatric symptoms including autism, and breast and colon cancer.

Dr. Galland has advanced the idea of four interlocking patterns of bacterial dysbiosis that pulls together all these ideas of pH into a modern paradigm explaining the physiological interactions we see and the pH connection to each.

Putrefaction

Dr. Galland says that putrefaction is the Western degenerative disease pattern that is the consequence of a diet high in fat and meat and low in fiber. A diet like this produces elevated concentrations of the bacterial species *Bacteroides sp.* and a decreased concentration of bifidobacteria in stools. It also provokes bacterial urease and beta-glucuronidase activity, ultimately resulting in abnormally alkaline colonic pH from excess ammonia in the colon. These bacterial enzymes may then metabolize bile acids, increasing tumors in the colon wall, and deconjugate estrogens in the stool, raising estrogen in the blood.

Dr. Galland believes that this type of dysbiosis contributes to colon cancer and breast cancer. He proposes that it be corrected by decreasing dietary fat and flesh, increasing fiber consumption, and using probiotics.

Excess Fermentation

Excess fermentation is a condition characterized by an excess of normal bacterial fermentation, usually resulting from bacterial overgrowth in the small intestine. It creates carbohydrate intolerance, with accompanying abdominal distention, flatulence, diarrhea, constipation, and general feelings of malaise.

Patients with fermentation excess usually do not tolerate soluble fiber supplements well, even though they are constipated and it would seem logical to try them. Dr. Galland suggests using antimicrobials and reducing carbohydrate consumption.

Deficiency

Previous use of antibiotics or a diet low in soluble fiber (conditions very common in modern Americans) may create a deficiency of normal stool bacteria, including bifidobacteria, lactobacilli, and *Escherichia coli* (*E. coli*). This is diagnosed by laboratory examination of the stool, to assess proper count of these good bugs. Irritable bowel syndrome and food intolerance are the result. The treatment for deficiency is the same as for putrefaction dysbiosis. Fructo-oligosaccharides are often helpful in reestablishing a normal flora.

Sensitization

In sensitization, the body develops an abnormal immune response to the toxins produced by normal intestinal flora. Treat sensitization by reestablishing normal body pH throughout the system and by long-term support of the immune system.

An Alkalinizing Daily Supplement Program

Since most Americans are too acid, we will concentrate on an alkalinizing supplement program. The following regime represents a consensus from the leading experts in the field and seems like a good basic program to raise pH to the proper alkaline level:

Bee pollen, according to label directions
Beta-carotene, 10,000 international units
Boron, 3 milligrams
Buffered vitamin C, 500 to 3,000 milligrams
Calcium, 800 to 1,500 milligrams
Chromium, 200 to 1,000 micrograms
Copper, 1 to 2 milligrams
Digestive enzymes with meals, according to label directions
Green superfoods (spirulina, chlorella, barley grass, wheat grass, chlorophyll), according to label directions
Iodine, 150 to 225 micrograms
Iron, 10 to 18 milligrams
Magnesium, 400 to 800 milligrams
Manganese, 10 to 30 milligrams
Nutritional yeast, according to label directions
Potassium, 99 to 300 milligrams
Royal jelly, according to label directions
Selenium, 50 to 200 micrograms
Vitamin B-complex, 50 milligrams
Zinc, 15 to 60 milligrams

All of these nutrients should be taken daily. The doses should be safe for long-term use. If desired, consult with your natural healing practitioner about good-quality brands and preparations.

Following this regime should gradually shift your body balance to normal. If you measure your urine periodically, you will gradually see a positive shift.

Exercise

Moderate aerobic exercise is important for everyone to maintain good health. It perks up circulation and increases oxygenation in the body. Breathing deeply brings more oxygen to all your tissues. It promotes a more alkaline pH.

If you are experiencing symptoms of excess acidity, you can up the effectiveness of your alkalinizing program by adding some sodium bicarbonate (baking soda) to your program, according to Dr. Lark. For other ways to use this substance, see "Vaginal Infection" on page 250.

Strenuous exercise such as running and heavy weight lifting causes your muscles to burn blood sugar and produce waste lactic and pyruvic acids. These acids produce muscle fatigue. As always, your body needs to buffer these potent acids. You can tell if you are flipping to the acid side when exercising if you get a slightly acidic taste in your mouth.

For a quick shot of alkaline, swallow a quarter to a half teaspoon of baking soda dissolved in a glass of water immediately after your workout to get yourself back in balance. By increasing the alkalinity of your blood, sodium bicarbonate buffers acidity in the muscles.

Some authorities take a dim view of this procedure, however. When you swallow baking soda, it goes first to your stomach, dissolving in the liquid stomach contents. This makes the stomach more basic. However, the stomach is supposed to be very acidic. Presumably the stomach then rebounds by producing more acid. So you can potentially end up either with inadequate acid for digesting food or with an overacid stomach and heartburn.

As it turns out, this might not be an issue if you wait to eat after drinking the baking soda mixture, Dr. Lark suggests. It is likely that the stomach can compensate for the temporary addition of the base and recover proper acidity before the next meal comes along. Wait half an hour after drinking the baking soda before eating.

Increasingly, physicians and scientists are recognizing the value of body balancing in their work with patients. Often, it's from seeing the results with their own eyes. Body pH is such a critical function that even an attempt to normalize functional chemistry meets with good success. Even professionals with conventional credentials are becoming converts. Slowly but surely, medical doctors and physiology experts are being exposed to the importance of pH chemistry and its role in recovering and maintaining good health. And these ideas really are sneaking into the mainstream.

Alternative practitioners are getting great results with very serious chronic conditions, including osteoporosis, heart disease, and arthritis—conditions that respond only to long, consistent health programs. Their patients, when they become conscious of their body's pH and begin to adjust, experience relief, often for the first time in years, from allergies, frequent colds, and acne. Holistic medicine has always held that the mind, the emotions, and the body are inseparable. Now we see that a missing link is body balancing. Scientific research has shown us that dietary change and supplementation, resulting in pH improvement, have profound effects on mind and behavior.

Body Balance is an innovative lens through which to view these wide-ranging health concerns. Natural healing in America has a history of being somewhat fragmented. But the historical systems on which it is based are very solid. Though they do not explicitly use pH, they all have a comprehensive system of understanding, evaluating, and restoring balance, as do the older systems from Europe and Asia including Ayurveda and TCM. When we add the modern understanding of pH to the puzzle, the underlying mechanisms and processes begin to come into focus. It seems as if the premises of the great healing systems, including American naturopathy, largely result in getting pH under control for the long run. Now we have the insight to understand what is happening from a chemical perspective, and a tool to monitor the changes in your body from day to day.

9

Body Balance Evaluation Techniques

It's quite clear that balancing pH and keeping it in balance are critical. But how will you know what the actual pH of your body fluids is? You'll test it, that's how. Scientists have come up with a variety of ways to evaluate the pH of your various juices, from a simple paper you dip in your saliva to a radio transmitter you swallow to assess your stomach acid. Many of these methods are easily available at a pharmacy or through the mail, but some require a doctor's consultation. Most you can accomplish privately at home.

Remember, the pH of your various body liquids varies considerably. Each liquid has it own special chemistry. Carefully study the proper pH range of the fluid you want to test, perform the test, and chart the measurement. If you are in the optimal range, congratulations. Then it's best to repeat the test a few times to make sure your pH for that fluid is consistent.

If you are out of range, which, unfortunately, we expect for most Americans, begin charting your measurements on a daily basis. In some cases, you might want to test and chart several times a day to assess the impact of meals or stress.

Tests for pH

What's the practical way to start down the path toward body balance? First you need to know where you stand. And to do that, you need to test the pH of each of your body fluids. A variety of tests are available, from simple paper strips you can use in your home to high-tech methods that are performed at a lab.

A good way to begin is to test the pH of your saliva and urine, both of which are easy to do. If you get the right type of strips, you can use them for both saliva and urine testing. Most pharmacies carry these. The paper is colored, and it will change color in a predictable way according to the acidity of the material with which it comes into contact. You read the pH by comparing the paper color to a gradated color chart.

Some packs contain individual, one-use strips, while other packages feature narrow pH paper on a continuous roll from which you need to tear off a piece to use each day. Most pH paper is very inexpensive. It comes in many configurations, though. You want a version that will read out a range from 5.0 (or 5.5) to 8.0, in gradations of 0.2, for accuracy.

Blood Tests

The body keeps the pH of the blood within an extremely narrow range. Arterial blood should be 7.35, while venous blood should be 7.46. Even a tiny deviation can be catastrophic. Since it is extremely rare to see blood pH changes, blood pH is not routinely measured. Home kits are not sensitive enough to be meaningful. Medical doctors can order such tests, but almost never do. The body will move heaven and earth to keep blood pH stable, including pumping the last reserves of alkaline minerals into the serum. So by the time the blood shows a deviation, things have gotten extremely serious and symptoms have shown up in other body systems. The fact remains, though, that the blood is the most important place for pH concern. The urine is already out of the body, and it reflects what has happened over a few hours.

About the only pH expert who tests blood pH is Dr. Harold J. Kristal, who has offices in San Rafael, California. Dr. Kristal is a dentist. He calls his approach "The Science of Metabolic Typing," which is sensibly based on the wisdom of treating the person who has the disease, instead of the disease that has the person.

Dr. Kristal claims that the importance for maintaining an optimal venous blood pH is absolutely critical, and he ultimately uses this measure as the bottom line for success. Any deviation can create lack of enzyme utilization, lack of trace nutrient absorption, and deficiencies in vitamins, minerals, and fatty acids. Obviously, since the blood pH varies so incredibly slightly, the equipment needed to measure it is complex and needs to be used in the practitioner's office. Along with other experts, Dr. Kristal claims that when these deviations are too great or go on for too long, degenerative and metabolic diseases—especially fatigue, digestive disorders, and allergies—manifest. He describes his methods in *The Nutrition Solution: A Guide to Your Metabolic Type* (North Atlantic Books, 2002).

Dr. Kristal maintains that many dietary schemes claim to promote energy and weight loss, but that they will work only in the long term if they are compatible with your metabolic type. One person can lose weight on a particular diet, but another person might gain weight on exactly the same program. Enter metabolic typing. It is the missing link that codifies why one person's food may literally be another person's poison.

Dr. Kristal and his associate, W. L. (Bill) Wolcott, have been working synergistically for the past two years and have jointly created a protocol to measure body chemistry. They conduct a fasting urine pH test, fasting blood glucose test, and a glucose tolerance test to determine the acid-alkaline biobalance profile. This procedure takes about one and a half hours and requires a fifteen-hour fast. Blood is drawn only from a lancet prick in the finger.

Dr. Kristal offers a home version of the test. The kit includes a glucose meter, test strips, pH papers, alcohol swabs, glucose and protein challenge powders, a self-test chart, a questionnaire, and a medical history form. The test is performed in your own home, on an empty stomach. After filling out the paperwork, you mail your results to Dr. Kristal for analysis. He provides you with the analysis of your metabolic type, along with recommendations regarding your diet and suggested supplements for your metabolism.

According to Dr. Kristal, there are five basic metabolic types. Two of them have the tendency to be too acid and need help to move their blood pH toward the alkaline side. Two have the tendency to be too alkaline and need to move more to the acid side. The final type tends to be close to the center, but may still need minor adjustments to move to the ideal balance. Dr. Kristal's wrinkle is that even if we know that the blood is too acid, we still don't know which foods will make it more alkaline. Unexpectedly, the reason is that any given food may be either alkalinizing or acidifying, depending on the metabolic type of the person ingesting it. Because of this, without some method of metabolic testing, effective nutritional protocols can happen only by chance, not through scientific rationale.

Dr. Kristal's five metabolic types are:

1. Fast oxidizer (acid blood)
2. Slow oxidizer (alkaline blood)
3. Sympathetic dominant (acid blood)
4. Parasympathetic dominant (alkaline blood)
5. Balanced/mixed

According to Dr. Kristal and other proponents of metabolic typing, the field of nutrition appears perplexing because what works for one patient with a specific condition does not work for a different patient with the same condition. The metabolic type, which is basically another way to express pH, is the key. For example, the slow oxidizer and the sympathetic dominant cannot tolerate a high-meat and -fat diet, but the fast oxidizer and the parasympathetic need just that in order to be healthy. And you can measure the progress with the ongoing tests.

Very few supplements are prescribed in Dr. Kristal's system. According to this protocol, the proper foods will nudge venous blood pH back into biobalance. When this adjustment occurs, great changes happen in your body. You will now absorb and utilize nutrients. When supplements are needed, it's important to remember that different supplements have diverse biochemical actions for each metabolic type. According to Dr. Kristal's finely tuned theory, potassium will acidify the blood in specific metabolic types (slow oxidizers) and alkalinize it in others (parasympathetics). Vitamin C is another case in point. Calcium ascorbate, which is alkaline forming in the blood, will alkalinize the blood; whereas ascorbic acid, being acid forming in the blood, will acidify the blood. Generally cancer patients' venous blood is alkaline. If these folks take the ascorbate form of vitamin C, it can further alkalinize their blood, reducing their ability to utilize many enzymes and trace nutrients.

Based on his career of testing pH and blood samples, Dr. Kristal says that the three major food categories causing health problems are vegetable oils that have been processed and refined into trans fatty acids and hydrogenated oils, refined sugars and grain products consumed in high quantities, and animal meats and animal fats consumed in high quantities. On the other hand, Dr. Kristal's three factors for optimizing health include a positive mental attitude, proper nutrition for your specific body chemistry, and adequate aerobic exercise for your age.

Saliva Tests

The pH of the saliva varies widely throughout the day, depending on what you eat. Saliva often rises to 7.8 or higher immediately after a meal. Salivary pH changes quickly, so several measurements need to be taken throughout the day to get a good average. Urine is a better guide, as it is a record of a few hours of accumulated metabolism.

It's simple to test your salivary pH at home using small paper strips. Get these at any pharmacy or from a supplier on the Internet. A good time to test saliva is upon arising, before putting anything in the mouth. Alternatively, you could wait for two hours after eating. Simply place a drop of saliva on the strip and read the color. Most strips are calibrated so that dark blue signifies alkalinity and yellow indicates acidity. With most kits, you will shoot for a medium green reading, right in the middle. Look for it to be in the ideal 6.0 to 7.0 range.

For a bit more money, you can get a reusable battery-operated pH meter. You can dip the tip into saliva and read the digital screen. Since paper is limited in range and also in accuracy, a meter is a much better long-term choice. If you can afford one, it will be a lifelong tool for you and your family.

There are many varieties of pH meters. Over the long run, meters with ISFET technology will have the longest life and require the least maintenance. Fitted with an electronic solid-state chip, this variety needs as little as one drop of fluid for testing. When the meter is calibrated carefully and used properly, your saliva (and urine) tests will be very accurate. This type of meter sells for about $235.

Cheaper meters with glass bulbs wear out fast, often require large sample sizes, and vary in accuracy depending on how well they are maintained.

To get a good average, engage in an ongoing test over several days, or even over a couple of weeks, to verify how your acidity fluctuates during the day under different circumstances and with different foods. Divide a piece of lined paper into five columns and label the columns "Time," "Foods," "Saliva pH," "Urine pH," and "Remarks." Starting first thing in the morning, record the time and your urine and saliva pH every time you urinate throughout the day. With each meal, record the time and what you eat. With each notation, make a comment about any symptoms, your mental state, and your level of energy.

Tracking what you eat, how it makes your pH respond, and how you feel can be an invaluable tool to begin to associate these factors. You will probably notice that every time you eat a certain food, your pH consistently goes in one direction a few hours later. You may start to notice patterns of mood, behavior, and energy that correspond to diet and pH. Now you are on the road to self-empowerment.

You can even challenge yourself to feel and see the difference with an experiment. Eat an acid-forming dinner. Tank up on meat, white pasta, fish, and sugar—but no vegetables! First thing in the morning, check your urine pH. In all likelihood, you will find the acid dumped, as it should be, in the urine, with a urine pH of from 4.5 up to 5.8 or so.

On the other hand, you could eat a test dinner of very alkaline foods—all vegetables. Again, check your first urine pH. A pH in the range of 6.8 to 8.5 means all is well and you are headed to that stable number of 6.4.

Urine Tests

Assessing the pH of your first morning urine is a good measure of average body pH. Urinate into a clean container, then dip in a one-inch-long strip of pH paper. Compare the resulting color with the chart that's included with the paper. If you find that your first morning urine is between 6.5 (slightly acidic) and 7.5 (slightly alkaline), it is a sign that your overall cellular pH is in balance. Even though it would seem that the more alkaline you are, the better, that's not true. When it comes to pH, it's all about balance. Urine pH can vary from 4.5 to 9.0 at the extremes, but urine numbers above 8.0 (alkaline) are a sign that your metabolism has become catabolic—that is, that it's destroying and consuming itself.

Some experts claim that urinary and salivary pH should remain pretty steady at 6.4 at all hours of the day. The idea is that variations from this "ideal" are caused by deficiencies in total alkaline reserves, allowing the pH to wobble. If the alkaline reserves are low enough so that they do not efficiently buffer the acid avalanche from eating, the saliva and urine pH will acidify for a while after a meal, thus prompting the variation to the acid side, especially in the saliva. According to this more conservative assessment, the longer and more vigorously we adjust our diet and lifestyle to build our alkaline reserves, the more we will experience a pH that is consistently stable and closer to the bull's eye of 6.4, the pH that seems to be the ideal for chemical reactions to be carried out in the body.

For a quick "average" pH assessment, measure the acidity of your urine and saliva two hours after breakfast and two hours after lunch. Over several days, average your numbers. Then add your average urine pH to the doubled average of your saliva pH, and divide the total by three. (The saliva figure is doubled in the averaging because it is more variable.) Apply this formula: (average urine pH + average saliva pH x 2) / 3 = average overall pH.

Let's take an example:

Average urine pH = 6.0
Average saliva pH = 7.0, multiplied by 2 = 14.0
6.0 + 14.0 = 20.0, divided by 3 = 6.7

The quick average pH comes out to 6.7.

As we discussed in Chapter 8, you can use this figure to assess your calcium need and choose the best type of calcium for your particular needs.

Your physician can order a noninvasive urine test that measures factors in the urine that are closely associated with bone mineral loss. It does not measure pH per se, but indicates the need for further action. Called the NTx test, it measures urinary excretion of cross-linked N-telopeptide of type I collagen.[1] It is offered by integrative gynecologists. You provide a sample of your second urine of the day. If it is out of normal, it might indicate calcium loss from bone, an inference of your possibly being at risk for osteoporosis. (For more on the NTx test, see page 110.)

A recent study measured the accuracy of the NTx test. The scientists concluded that urinary NTx does represent changes in bone metabolism caused by estrogen deficiency and that it may be a more sensitive and specific marker than other common tests in the early postmenopausal years.[2]

Heidelberg Test

Physicians evaluate the stomach's capacity to produce acid secretions with the Heidelberg test, which uses a radiotelemetry capsule.[3,4,5] The Heidelberg gastrogram was created by researchers in Heidelberg, Germany, during the mid-1960s.

The patient swallows a small plastic capsule (about the size of an extra-strength aspirin) containing electronic monitoring equipment. The capsule measures the pH of the stomach, small intestine, and large intestine. Transmitting a signal to an external receiver, the capsule provides information on the pH of the active digestive organs.

When the capsule reaches the stomach, the pH is recorded. If normal, the stomach's ability to secrete hydrochloric acid on demand may be challenged by having the patient drink a small quantity of sodium bicarbonate (baking soda), a highly alkaline substance. This should bring the pH back up to 8.0 or so. A healthy stomach should then be able to acidify the solution within ten to fifteen minutes. The alkaline solution may be given up to four times, each time after the stomach has been reacidified. If the stomach is incapable of this repeated reacidification, the physician may make a diagnosis of hypochlorhydria. Short-term treatment of hypochlorhydria may include supplementing with highly acidic betaine hydrochloride or glutamic acid with meals.

The capsule can be attached to a string and recovered by pulling it out, or it will be allowed to pass in a normal bowel movement.

Tests to determine the pH of the stomach contents can also be performed by aspirating stomach liquid through a tube inserted down the throat or by vomiting.

Nutri-Spec

Chanchal Cabrera, M.N.I.M.H., A.H.G., is a widely respected herbalist. A member of the prestigious Institute of Medical Herbalists in England, she has had a high profile in the world of clinical herbal medicine. She is the author of *Fibromyalgia: A Journey Toward Healing* (McGraw-Hill, 2002).

According to the system she recommends, which is called Nutri-Spec, no two people are alike. Each person's physical, mental, and emotional qualities are an indication of individual body chemistry. Each person is built differently and has different requirements. This concept of biological individuality, including pH, gives us a new way to look at nutrition. This system measures a set of parameters in the individual and identifies *a pattern of dysfunction*, defined by a collection of aberrant test results. These deviations indicate loss of homeostasis.

According to the Nutri-Spec system, every condition can be defined in terms of its *patterns of metabolic imbalance*. Rather than naming and treating a *disease*, the *pattern* (including pH) is defined and treated. This is a patient-specific approach, based on biological individuality.[6]

Nutri-Spec uses tests of urine and saliva chemistries and tests of vital signs and neuroendocrine reflexes. The method calculates five factors in the urine and saliva analysis, including pH, parasympathetic-sympathetic ratio, aerobic-anaerobic ratio, hydration (electrolyte balance), and glucogenic-ketogenic ratio (whether you re getting cell fuel from sugars or fats). These ratios indicate how to individualize the diet and supplementation program.

Self-Test for Stomach pH

As an alternative to a laboratory test such as the Heidelberg capsule test, some practitioners have their patients test their own stomach acid levels. This subjective test is less accurate than the Heidelberg test, but it is convenient and inexpensive. On the first day, the patient takes one 10-grain (650-milligram) tablet of betaine hydrochloride in tablet form. If any discomfort, nausea, or burning occurs, we can conclude that the stomach is already acidic enough and no further supplementation is necessary. If the challenge is comfortable, the patient continues to take one tablet with each meal for the rest of the day.

On successive days, the patient increases the per-meal dose by one tablet. Once any tickling or burning sensation is noted, the per-meal dose is reduced by one tablet and continued as a supplemental way to temporarily acidify the stomach.

People should not take hydrochloric acid tablets along with anything that might irritate the stomach lining, such as aspirin, cortisone, or a similar drug. Hydrochloric acid supplements should not be chewed. The acid can harm the teeth.

Reams Technique

Carey Reams was a chemist working earlier in the twentieth century. While he was not a credentialed physician in the United States, he worked with a modern scientific model. He did some of the critical work on pH in the century. He developed pH tests of blood, urine, and saliva and created an interpretive system for the results, as well as treatment protocols. Reams did not write much, but he taught many people. His work has been carried on in seminars and is used by a cadre of present-day physicians.

Reams, a self-proclaimed biophysicist, was called a physician by some, although he did not have medical credentials. He was prosecuted during the 1970s for practicing medicine without a license. About fifty years ago, he developed the Reams Biological Theory of Ionization.

During World War II, Reams was severely injured in a landmine explosion that left him a quadriplegic. Later, he attended a faith-healing service that apparently produced a miraculous cure. Reams's subsequent conversion to Christianity greatly colored his later work, as he came to see nature as divinely ordered and holistic.

Reams was originally an agricultural biochemist. He developed an outstanding reputation for being able to work wonders with the soil. He applied his talents mainly to golf course owners having turf trouble and to farmers with crop problems.

Reams's dual interests in agriculture and medicine contributed to his understanding of a link between human health and soil health. The concept that human health problems are directly related to the mineral depletion of our soil was becoming popular. Reams worked with the concepts of the day and demonstrated the efficacy of these principles. Reams's clients grew crops that were disease-free and resistant to pests. Eventually, Reams established a health retreat in the Blue Ridge Mountains of Georgia, where people would come for several weeks and be given a diet to suit their body chemistry.

Reams had adapted a soil- and plant-testing technique to test urine and saliva. The procedure involves standard soil-testing tools. The analysis is derived from seven basic metabolic parameters in the urine and saliva. The test yields valuable information on the efficiency of the digestive system and immune system, as well as specific information on what vitamins and minerals are not being assimilated into the body's cellular structure.

The Reams technique is a simple, noninvasive test that an individual can do in less than ten minutes. The test includes the seven parameters of body chemistry. The evaluation procedures are all performed on samples of saliva and urine. Reams said he was guided by God to develop a mathematical formula for perfect health, based on the biophysical frequencies of living matter. After extensive research, Reams discovered the "perfect numbers" for Biological Ionization, his term for the collected processes of metabolism, which represent the ideal cellular conditions required for life. Reams theorized that the seven parameters, all normalized simultaneously, represent the perfect 100-percent conversion of food into energy. The idea is that if a person could maintain a lifestyle that maintained the "perfect numbers," he or she would not experience premature aging.

The test collection (seven parameters) consists of sugar (sometimes referred to as carbohydrate level), urine pH, saliva pH, conductivity (sometimes referred to as salt content, important because salt increases electrical conductivity), cell debris (sometimes referred to as albumen), nitrate nitrogen, and ammonia nitrogen.

The test series is designed to reveal the calcium needs of your particular body chemistry, digestive efficiency, nutrient assimilation, vitamin and mineral deficiencies, blood sugar status, immune function, and major organ (kidneys, liver, heart, colon, and gallbladder) function. After the initial testing, the analysis is often repeated every one to four weeks to assess progress.

The Seven Parameters of Reams

The sugar (or carbohydrate) measurement of the Reams technique indicates the amount of potential energy available per pound of body weight or, said another way, carbohydrate utilization. It is made with a refractometer, an instrument used in wine making and soil testing, and measures sugar content in brix units, a unit of sugar content used in agriculture. The ideal carbohydrate measure is 1.5 brix. A medium healing range is 1.2 to 2.0 brix. Below 1.2 represents low blood sugar, and above 5.5 represents borderline diabetes. Reams proponents use this measure, in relationship to the other parameters, to get an idea about vitamin C metabolism, headache patterns, alcohol levels, body temperature, alertness, seizure potential, and morning sickness.

According to the Reams system, the two-part test of pH indicates the speed at which energy is moving through the body. It measures how well the body is using energy and eliminating what is left over after digestion—in other words, whether we are putting in enough energy to replace what we are taking out. A reading of 6.4 is the ideal for saliva and urine. Urine pH supplies information about the blood and the efficiency of the kidneys in removing toxins from the body and juices of the stomach, while salivary pH indicates the condition of the liver and pancreatic enzymes. The pH test involves testing urine and saliva with pH paper that measures pH in two-tenths increments or a pH meter twice a day for three days.

This analysis of pH gives an overview of digestive speed and indigestion, calcium needs and type, calcium levels, insulin functions, microbial infection susceptibility, and vitamin C and B_{12} levels.

An acceptable range in a healing person is 6.2 to 6.6. According to the Reams system, you add your urine pH number to two times your saliva pH number and divide by three to obtain your average bodily pH.

The test of urine mineral salts provides information on the electrical conductance of the body fluids. It is essentially a measure of electrolyte balance. It is done using a standard conductivity meter. Conductivity testers measure the electrical conductivity (EC) of water, soil, compost, and in this case, urine. EC is measured in micro Siemens. In the Reams test, 700 micro Siemens equal 1 salt unit. The ideal reading is 6 to 7 salt units.

The urine salt level reveals the body fluid balance, rate of tissue breakdown, cholesterol level, and condition of the heart, blood vessels, nerves, and muscles.

The cell debris (sometimes called albumen) test is a measure of the number of dead cells leaving the body, a reflection of cellular breakdown from pathology. The ideal cell debris number is 0.04, or 4 million particles per liter of urine. The cell debris number reflects the speed of the body's healing process. As the body ages, it needs to heal itself. A lot of daily healing is a sign that a large amount of tissue is breaking down and that aging is too rapid. A high cell debris number therefore indicates that the body is using up too much of its resources to run too fast—that is, burning too much fuel to maintain an elevated body temperature and too rapid metabolism. Running fast causes stress (premature aging) on the tissues, resulting in damage and cellular debris. The body then needs to expend extra energy to heal the damaged tissues.

The cell debris number is the last of the Reams numbers to come into balance because the body continues to heal damage from the past even as the other fluids become properly adjusted chemically. You can get a pretty good idea of the albumen level of urine by holding up a sample of the urine in front of a light. The urine should be clear. A cloudy appearance indicates a high albumen level. Cell debris tests reveal kidney stresses, energy loss, and the need for vitamins E, A, and C.

Urine ammonia and nitrates should each be 3.0. When added together and taken as one value, the figure is the total ureas, measured in the urine. This measurement shows how well we digest protein and whether we are eating too much protein. It also indicates how well the large and small intestines conduct their eliminative functions. Total ureas correspond to the amount of unutilized protein that is being processed by the liver and sent to the kidneys for elimination. It is also an indication of protein digestion potential, protein/nitrogen/meat toxicity or deficiency, potassium uptake and dumping, bile salt strength, and thyroid status.

A total greater than 6 (the sum of both nitrogen figures) indicates an excess of urea, the by-product of protein digestion in the blood. (From our previous discussion, we know that protein breakdown produces acid, so we would expect to see this along with an increased acid pH.) Reams said that pork, rabbit, and mollusks in the diet can up this number. High urea can be caused by not drinking enough water. Common warning signs of high urea include fatigue after a normal amount of sleep and deep forehead wrinkles from anxiety.

Reams's Remedies

To combat the warning signs of high urea and restore proper body balance, Reams developed a thorough regime of diet and lifestyle changes that individualized his therapy for the patient. He was a proponent of detoxification procedures. He used herbs, minerals, and a variety of other supplements for body biochemical balancing, and he included simple lymphatic exercises.

After testing hundreds of substances, Reams found that fresh lemons and liver bile had the greatest number of characteristics he was seeking to balance the most people efficiently. Reams advocated drinking plenty of lemon water for pH balance, enhanced liver function, and general nutrition. He sought to increase liver bile production by adjusting the diet. He found that calcium, potassium, and chlorine have these benefits, too.

He said that calcium deficiency in the liver reduces the bile in the body, thus affecting the pH balance. He proposed drinking half of the body weight in ounces of water each day. For example, a person weighing 100 pounds should drink 50 ounces of water daily.

Comprehensive Digestive Stool Analysis

Let's face it, dinner table discussion it's not. But your large intestine is every bit as important as your other less unsavory body parts.

One way we can get an idea of the health of the colonic digestive processes is to assess fecal pH. This measurement appears to be a pretty good indicator of the health status of that area. Many alternative physicians use cutting-edge laboratory tests. The Great Smokies Diagnostic Laboratory specializes in the medical tests requested by more avant garde doctors.[7] One of the diagnostic panels it offers is the Comprehensive Digestive Stool Analysis (CDSA), which evaluates a stool sample for a number of important parameters that tell us about body balance, including pH, digestion, triglycerides, chymotrypsin, iso-butyrate, iso-valerate, n-valerate, meat and vegetable fibers, absorption, long-chain fatty acids, cholesterol, total fecal fat, and total short-chain fatty acids.

It's also important to check the microbe levels in the stool. The Great Smokies test includes microbiology (levels of lactobacilli, bifidobacteria, *E. coli*, and other "potential pathogens," including *Aeromonas, Bacillus cereus, Campylobacter, Citrobacter, Klebsiella, Proteus, Pseudomonas, Salmonella, Shigella, Staphylococcus aureus,* and *Vibrio*) and identification and quantification of fecal yeast (including *Candida albicans, C. tropicalis, Rhodotorula,* and *Geotrichum*).

Other important factors are also included. The test covers n-butyrate (considered a key energy source for colonic epithelial cells), beta-glucuronidase, short-chain fatty acid distribution (adequate amounts and proportions of the different short-chain fatty acids reflect the basic status of the intestinal metabolism), immunology, and fecal secretory immunoglobulin A (a measure of immunologic function).

The results are reported individually or combined into a "dysbiosis risk index," which is a calculation based on the net value of the gut microbiology, pH, and short-chain fatty acids.

Elevated fecal triglycerides suggest pancreatic insufficiency. High amounts of iso-butyrate, iso-valerate, and n-valerate (short-chain fatty acids) reflect the presence of undigested protein in the bowel. This is due to either eating too much protein or not metabolizing it well enough. Long-chain fatty acids (free fatty acids) in the stool indicate malabsorption. Elevated fecal cholesterol is abnormal and may indicate malabsorption.

The CDSA helps identify gut imbalances, supplies clues about confusing symptoms, and identifies areas that could be problematic should the imbalances progress. After such an assessment, a treatment plan can be custom tailored, greatly increasing the chances for therapeutic success.

Biological Terrain Assessment

Biological Terrain Assessment (BTA) is a technique used by many holistic physicians. The method uses a computerized measurement system developed by naturopathic physician and chiropractor Robert Greenberg that assesses the characteristics of the blood, urine, and saliva, including pH, and plots the results on a software grid. Physicians can see the early signs of a disease at the cellular level before the disease manifests. Based on this analysis, they can determine the underlying metabolic imbalances and prescribe dietary changes and remedial supplements.

"If in checking we find that your cellular chemistry—biological terrain—is going astray, we know that your entire cellular functioning will soon follow, resulting in illness," Dr. Greenberg explains. "This enables us to then start correcting the imbalance using natural means, such as nutrition, supplements, or homeopathy, among others, before your condition becomes pathological and requires more invasive medical procedures." The key point here, he says, is that terrain assessment "gives you the ability to see if the patient's chemistry is running optimally, even if he is not experiencing any symptoms."

The term "bioterrain" refers to the environment in which all living things exist. Each type of living organism requires different conditions (such as temperature, pH, and food) for optimal functioning. If we can live within our optimal range, our ability to live and effectively reproduce is improved. This is our "bioterrain."

Friendly bacteria (such as acidophilus, bifidus, and bulgaricus), which thrive naturally in the human body, prefer a similar bioterrain. These bacteria are necessary to our health in many ways. Some of them increase nutrient absorption in the gut. Some help us to fight off harmful microbes. According to proponents of the bioterrain idea, these bugs grow much better in a slightly alkaline environment.

Harmful invaders such as viruses, bacteria, fungi, molds, parasites, and yeast function at their best in a slightly different bioterrain. If the human body moves away from its ideal bioterrain and slips toward the bioterrain that these "bad bugs" prefer, it will eventually succumb to disease.

Bad bugs prefer a more acidic pH, which is another reason to keep your pH on the alkaline side.

If your intracellular pH swings to a more acidic state, you may witness the beginning of a series of unhealthy processes—a "pH cascade." The bad bugs will multiply.

Increased free radical activity, caused in part by environmental toxins such as secondhand smoke, a meal high in saturated fats, or extreme stress, causes your bioterrain to become significantly damaged. Again your bioterrain becomes more acidic, causing the development of more "bad bugs."

Like ungracious house guests, the "bad bugs" themselves give off acidic toxins, creating just the acid soup they so prefer. And the vicious circle continues.

The excess acidity causes cellular damage, or more free radicals. An accompanying lack of antioxidants allows the free radicals to race around, slamming into cell membranes, possibly ultimately damaging the cells' DNA and RNA molecules.

According to BTA proponents, in general, the urine is a better indicator of pH changes than is the blood. The blood's pH level is very tightly controlled. However, if we look at both measures together and take salivary pH into account, we can get a more complete picture of the body's chemical balance.

This school of thought claims that urine is a good indicator of the body's secretory ability and toxic cell load, while blood is a good indicator of toxicity and oxygen balance. Saliva gives a clue to a person's digestive capacities. Taken together and monitored over time, these factors provide a benchmark for determining whether a person's health is improving or slipping.

Physicians practicing according to this philosophy say that the pH measurement can not only determine if a patient's biochemistry is too acidic or too alkaline, but can indicate whether the enzymatic activity in the body is taking place appropriately and if the digestion and absorption of vitamins, minerals, and other nutrients is satisfactory. They can also infer from this procedure the presence of environmental and industrial contaminants.

It's tremendously important to have a fundamental understanding of the state of your body chemistry. By getting a baseline reading, you will be able to discern whether you are making progress as you engage in your Body Balance program. Start by testing some of your body fluids. You can do most of these tests at home, or you can have your holistic practitioner order them for you.

Once you know the lay of the land, it's time to get to work. Using the methods discussed in this book, you can begin to adjust your lifestyle, diet, and supplement program. The nice thing about pH testing is that its shows the results of your efforts pretty quickly. You will know if you are going in the right direction when you see your pH reading. Each test will have a target goal. As you begin to shift toward a more balanced pH, you will know whether you are making the progress you want, at the speed you want. If things need to be nudged along a bit faster, you can get down to it with a bit more diligence and a positive attitude.

Use the changes you experience in your body's pH to motivate you. Many people have gone through these changes before you and are now enjoying the benefits. They all say they wouldn't go back. Keep up with your discipline and soon, healthy living will be a way of life—the Body Balance way of life!

10

Food and Diet

Diet is probably the aspect of life that has the biggest impact on health. Let's face it: We do a lot of eating in our four score and ten. It's also likely that for most people, it's the thing that we have done the worst for the longest. It seems like it's all too easy to put off till tomorrow what we could do today. One more day won't hurt. Right?

Actually, one more day *won't* hurt. It's the 3,000 "one more" days strung together that add up. So, can we approach food and diet in a rational way, in a way that will be possible to do and that will get results? Yes.

In this chapter, we will look at the ins and outs of body balance with food. We'll start with the basics, such as taste, and work our way into the details of a healthy, pH-balancing diet. On our journey to a healthier kitchen, we will review the major food types and how to evaluate and adjust their effects, good and bad. Finally, we'll put it all together with a collection of delicious yet convenient recipes.

Taste

Taste is a quick and valuable way to determine the probable action of an herb or food. Remember that all the macronutrients (carbohydrates, proteins, and fats) have a sweet taste. They all increase the acid load. So, for most people, the fewer sweet-tasting foods, the better.

Ayurveda says that salty taste is heating. TCM says that salty taste is cooling. And they are both right.

Remember, minerals generally taste salty, so cooling, alkalinizing calcium is included with heating, acidifying chlorine. Ayurveda has observed that table salt quickens the metabolism and improves digestion, which are heating effects. TCM focuses on the fact that table salt contains sodium and promotes water retention, which is a cooling effect.

According to Dr. Michael Tierra:

> Energetics between different traditional systems is not a rational or strict thing, so one cannot look at traditional designations as one might view a scientific study. To truly understand the energetics of complex and great systems such as TCM and Ayurveda, one must look more deeply into the traditional classifications and try to understand from the perspective of that system why something such as salt is classified as heating in Ayurveda or cooling in TCM. One clue is that initially salt is irritating and will cause an immediate heating reaction. From the TCM perspective, salt is a mineral, so it is cool, but more important, it promotes fluid retention, which is yin, which is classified as cooling.

Have you ever eaten something that was way too salty? Perhaps you put too much salt on your popcorn at the movie theater. Did you have heartburn shortly after eating it? That effect is from the chlorine in the salt. When salt hits the liquid in your stomach, the salt molecule disassociates into a sodium ion and a chlorine ion. Some of the chlorine combines with the hydrogen in the water of your stomach, forming hydrochloric acid: instant acid heartburn. Chlorine is an acid mineral that drives overall pH down.

Balancing pH with Food

We've talked extensively about the fact that most Americans are too acidic. However, what is true for one individual may not be true for another. Your specific situation might not be the norm. You might be a natural high-alkaline producer. Perhaps you grew up in another culture with a different diet. Perhaps you are one of the lucky ones with a lower stress load. You might have been living right, whether by accident or by design, and be in balance, or even too alkaline, right now.

Remember that our goal is balance. You are an individual, and you need to treat yourself as an individual. Perhaps you, in fact, are one of the few high-alkaline persons. You can afford to, and probably should, use more acid foods in your diet.

There have been a few attempts to classify people into groups based on their physiology. These methods rely on some measures of metabolism, such as hair or blood mineral profiles or blood types. These schemes divide the public into groups along a spectrum, essentially along pH line. A scheme using four groups might be divided as follows:

1. High acid
2. Low acid
3. Low alkaline
4. High alkaline

Some people, therefore, can consume more acid-producing foods than others. Hunter-gatherers consuming salt-free diets rich in fruits and vegetables have demonstrated a high immunity to age-related degenerative diseases. Scientists at the University of California, San Francisco, analyzed known hunter-gatherer diets for net endogenous acid production (NEAP). They compared their total acid load with that of contemporary diets, which are typified by an imbalance of nutrient precursors of hydrogen and bicarbonate. This induces a lifelong, low-grade, pathogenical metabolic acidosis. After studying 159 preagricultural diets, they determined that 87 percent were net alkaline producing. The shift from negative to positive NEAP was accounted for by the reduction of the high-bicarbonate-yielding plant foods that had been in the ancestral diet and their replacement by cereal grains and energy-dense, nutrient-poor foods in the modern diet. The researchers reported that diet-induced metabolic acidosis reflects a mismatch between the nutrient composition of the current diet and the genetically determined nutritional requirements for optimal systemic acid-alkaline balance.[1]

The people of rural Crete (eating the so-called Mediterranean diet) have very low recorded rates of degenerative diseases—and they live a long time. Their daily diet incorporates about 2 pounds of fresh fruits and vegetables. But here's the rub: It includes only 1 pound of grain products; 3 ounces of meat, fish, and eggs; and 1 ounce of legumes. All those vegetables and fruits make this a neutral or slightly alkaline diet.

In the final analysis, you need to treat yourself with common sense and compassion. Do what you can. Use the techniques in this book to determine where you are, personally, along the pH spectrum. Then build your own therapeutic diet from there.

Nutrients in an Alkalinizing Diet Program

Essential fatty acids (EFAs) are building blocks for hormonelike chemicals called prostaglandins. There are many prostaglandins produced by the body. Some are beneficial, and yet others provoke damaging responses, including inflammation. Dr. Lark says that the series one prostaglandin PGE prevents inflammation, reducing the symptoms of arthritis. Fatty acids are incorporated into cartilage and bone. They make up the main structural component of all cell membranes. Your brain, nerves, retina, adrenal glands, skin, and mucous membranes particularly need EFAs. In fact, fats compose more than 60 percent of your brain.

Essential fatty acids are not specifically alkalinizing. In fact, they might actually be slightly acidifying. However, they contribute to the level of anti-inflammatory prostaglandins helping to reverse the inflammatory damage caused by acidosis.[2]

Whole, unrefined foods generally contain some EFAs. Whole grains and seeds are especially rich sources. Dietary supplement sources of EFAs include evening primrose oil, black currant seed oil, and flaxseed oil.

Dietary oils that have been extracted from seeds and nuts, including almond, sesame, and olive, can be economical and excellent sources of beneficial EFAs. Focus on getting whole, unrefined, cold-pressed oils. Commercial sources tend to have problems with quality, though. In many, the EFAs have been damaged by exposure to heat, light, or air, so make sure you buy a good-quality product. An excellent book on this subject is *Fats That Heal, Fats That Kill* by Udo Erasmus (Alive Books, 1993).

In *The pH Miracle* (Warner Books, 2002), Robert O. Young, Ph.D., claims that ghee (clarified butter) and coconut oil are the least acidifying dietary fats.[3] Ayurveda specifically calls these two fats the most cooling (anti-inflammatory) of all.

Even better, skip the processing and eat the raw seeds and nuts as food. Flax, sesame, sunflower, pumpkin, pecan, and walnut are superb sources of fatty acids. Avocado is rich in healthy monounsaturated fats, potassium, and protein.

If you consume flesh, fish—salmon, trout, and tuna, for instance—are good sources of the anti-inflammatory EFAs.

Surprisingly, green leafy vegetables are sources of fatty acids. Even though the percentage they contain is tiny, it is easy to eat large quantities of this tasty chow.

What About Meat, Fish, and Protein?

The consensus of the authorities who are proponents of the acid-balancing method of healthcare is that the vast majority of Americans are too acid. Dr. Robin Dipasquale maintains that, on the whole, the American culture eats too much protein. This may or may not be true in any other particular country. We have discussed some examples of other cultures and their diets and the results they experience.

But every country has a different set of circumstances. Diets vary, of course, but so do ethnic history, geography, and economics. It's a big job to sort it all out. Modern science is getting off to a good start, and we have identified some excellent major concepts from large studies of diets in different countries. For example, we now know that green tea, consumed largely in Asia, is an important health promoter.

Authorities differ in their attitude toward animal flesh in the diet. Moral issues aside, red meat is a rich source of many nutrients. It is almost pure protein, and it is high in iron, a mineral that may be more difficult to come by in a vegetarian diet. The real problem has been the excessive quantity of low-quality meat that Americans have been increasingly eating over the past century. The experts quoted in this book all pretty much suggest that Americans should focus on alkalinizing. But nothing is ever that easy, is it?

Some physicians feel that reasonable amounts of quality meat protein have a role to play in maintaining health. Others point out the value of a vegetarian diet.

Alan Gaby, M.D., is one of the preeminent holistic physicians in the United States. A professor at Bastyr University in Seattle, he is the author of many professional publications for physicians, as well as *Preventing and Reversing Osteoporosis: What You Can Do About Bone Loss* (Prima Publishing, 1995). Dr. Gaby mentions that a vegetarian diet has been shown to reduce osteoporosis.

Dr. Dipasquale confirms that animal products promote acid pH, but she also reminds us that each body is unique and that there are other factors at play in addition to acid-base balance.

But wait. Is something afoul here? Chicken: the flesh health nuts love to recommend. Ideas are all over the place on this one. It is clearly less acid producing than red meat, but to what degree no one can agree. It probably lies somewhere between beef and fish. So why make a flap over it?

Dr. Brown maintains, "Meat is fine. It just has to be balanced by more potassium, found in vegetables, at least two servings each at lunch and dinner, so that the pH balance is maintained. The average American can buffer about 50 to 60 grams per day of protein. Most are eating well over that, and 100 grams per day is common."

Dr. Brown mentions that the recently popularized Paleolithic diet does include more meat than most Americans currently eat, but that proponents of this approach claim that it actually is an alkalinizing diet on balance because it incorporates a very large amount of high-potassium fruits and vegetables.

From the pH point of view, fish flesh may be less evil. Dr. Lark, even while suggesting eliminating red meat, points out that fish is less acidic and contains the beneficial anti-inflammatory oils. In her program, she includes it as an alternative to red meat as a source of protein.

Fish is acid producing—just less so than red meat. Depending on where you fall along the pH spectrum, you can make a decision about whether, and how much, to include in your diet.

Which Foods Are Which, Anyway?

Each tissue in the body has a pH at which it functions most efficiently. The stomach, for example, is very acid, and it is supposed to be that way. The gallbladder, on the other hand, is quite alkaline—again, for a reason. We are talking about the overall balance of acidity in the body as a whole. Sometimes it is even necessary to increase the pH in one organ while reducing the pH in another. In fact, in our culture, this is quite common. Skilled practitioners are trained in how to accomplish this. For our purposes, we are attempting to restore the balance of the body overall.

Since the concept of pH was formalized only in the early part of the twentieth century and many of these naturopathic dietary principles have been around for thousands of years, experts are still trying to sort it all out. People of goodwill can disagree on a few details, but they tend to be remarkably consistent on the major themes.

Any given two authorities might disagree about whether a specific fruit becomes slightly acid or slightly alkaline when ultimately digested. However, they all are in accord about the bad effects of the standard American diet (tellingly abbreviated SAD) of low vegetable and low fiber content.

Also, any given food can be good for you in one way and not so good for you in another way. That's where tailoring these programs to you as an individual comes in. That's the specialty of systems like Ayurveda and TCM. For example, many people consider yogurt to be the ultimate health food. There is certainly considerable folklore about its benefits and a corresponding amount of scientific literature promoting it. This book mentions beneficial probiotics several times. Yet most authorities consider yogurt to add to the body's acid load. It certainly has an acid pH when it is measured in a bowl. Yogurt contains organic acids. It is sour. Ayurveda has said for centuries that people with high pitta (read acid) should not eat yogurt. Even though the probiotics help the gut, for some people, the food as a whole is just too acid.

The Metabolic pH Effects of Foods

So now that we've talked a lot about pH and food, it's time to actually eat something. Instead of hauling a supercomputer to the store to calculate pH values, see Table 10.1. If, like most Americans, you are on the acid side, choose mainly foods from the alkaline side of the table and eschew the foods on the acid side. If you are one of the rare alkaline cases, select your diet more from the acid side of the table. The neutral foods are okay for everyone, should you wish to consume them.

The foods appearing in Table 10.1 may be good or bad for you in other ways, however. The chart is just to point you in the right direction if you are working to adjust your net pH balance. Also, recall that authorities may disagree about the specific effect of any given food. The net effect is the key. Do the best you can and monitor the benefits. If what you are doing is working, you don't need to get caught up in the details.

Echoing the Ayurvedic perspective, Dr. Dipasquale affirms that it is the *postdigestive* effect that is the key. But this is not necessarily the pH

Table 10.1. Acid, Alkaline, and Neutral Foods

Acid Foods	Mild or Neutral Foods	Alkaline Foods
	Meat and Protein Substitutes	
Chicken Eggs Red meat (beef, pork) Seafood (lobster, oyster)	Fish	Tofu
	Vegetables	
Concentrated, cooked tomato sauce (pizza sauce)	Acorn squash Butternut squash Dried beans (kidney, lima, mung, navy, pinto, soy, white) Eggplant Lentil Potato Pumpkin Sweet potato Yam	Artichoke Asparagus Avocado Beet and beet greens Bell pepper Cabbage Carrot Cauliflower Celery Chard Cilantro Cucumber Garlic Grasses (such as wheat grass) Green beans Kohlrabi Leek Lettuce Lotus root Okra Onion Parsley Peas Radish Rutabaga Spinach Sprouts Taro root Tomato Turnip Watercress Zucchini

Table 10.1. Acid, Alkaline, and Neutral Foods (Continued)

Acid Foods	Mild or Neutral Foods	Alkaline Foods
	Fruit	
Apple		Banana
Apricot		Coconut
Cranberry		Fig
Grape		Grapefruit
Mango		Lemon
Melon		Lime
Orange		Nectarine
Papaya		Persimmon
Peach		Sweet berries
Pear		
Pineapple		
Plum		
Sour berries		
Tangerine		
	Grains	
White flour	Amaranth	Brown rice
White rice	Kamut	Buckwheat
	Oat	Millet
	Quinoa	Spelt
	Whole wheat	
	Milk Products	
Cheese	Butter	
Yogurt	Ghee	
	Milk	
	Nuts, Seeds, and Legumes	
Peanut	Sesame seed	Almond
		Brazil nut
		Cashew
		Pumpkin seed

Table 10.1. Acid, Alkaline, and Neutral Foods (Continued)		
Acid Foods	**Mild or Neutral Foods**	**Alkaline Foods**
	Condiments	
Jelly with added sugar	Honey	Apple cider vinegar
Lard	Most oils (avocado, coconut,	Ginger root
	olive, pumpkin seed)	Miso
	Rice syrup	Molasses
	Sea salt	Seaweeds
		Soy sauce
	Beverages	
Carbonated drinks	Green tea	Mineral water
Fruit juices		Vegetable juices
	Miscellaneous	
		Baking soda

that is measured with litmus paper when the food is in a bowl. The post-digestive effect of any food or herb must be determined by years, or even generations, of experience. That is how several experts can claim that lemon, while acid outside the body, has a net alkalinizing effect when eaten.

Authorities Disagree

Even the most educated and committed experts can disagree about details. So, as you would expect, there are some bones (or should we say tofu slices?) of contention. First on the disagreement docket: citrus fruits, especially lemons. Though lemon has a very acid pH when compared to other fruits, Aihara classifies it as very yin. Most experts call lemons, limes, and grapefruits alkalinizing. These fruits contain very little sugar, reducing the fermentation that produces acid. Dr. Brown says that weak food acids (including citric acid) are converted to weak bases in the body, and that apple cider vinegar is also a good source of a weak base. To test this in your body, eat a large serving of one of these citrus fruits and then test your pH a while later.

Tomato also might be a problem. Acid in pH before being eaten, tomato produces alkaline reactions in the body. This is probably because it has little natural sugar, a substance well known as a big problem for acid. Aihara calls wine alkaline forming. Others disagree. Even though anyone who has ever had a cup of coffee might think this liquid is acid, Aihara says that coffee is alkaline forming. Almost all other authorities strongly disagree. Coffee has a pH of about 5.0, so it's closer to neutral than many of the acid fruits, but when compared to pH readings of over 6.0 for grains and close to 6.0 for many vegetables, coffee may be too acid for many. Also, it contains caffeine. A recent study done by researchers from the Bone Metabolism Unit of Creighton University's School of Medicine found that elderly women with high caffeine intakes showed much higher rates of spinal bone loss than those with low intakes. Low tissue vitamin D levels made it worse. The researchers looked at several risk factors, including calcium intake, caffeine intake, and smoking. The factor that had the most severe effect was caffeine intake. Researchers reported that taking in more than 300 milligrams per day of caffeine (the amount in about three cups of coffee) accelerated bone loss in elderly postmenopausal women.[4]

Dr. Lark and Dr. Brown applaud nuts as a source of protein that is less acid than meat. But Aihara calls nuts acid forming, probably just because they are protein sources and, as we now know, all protein breaks down into acid by-products. Sulfur-containing vegetables, particularly from the cabbage family, which includes cauliflower, Brussels sprouts, broccoli, and cabbage, might be a problem for some people. Sulfur is an acid-producing mineral. On the other hand, these vegetables also contain other alkaline nutrients. The onion family, which also includes garlic and chives, is high in sulfur, as well. Dr. Dipasquale says olive oil, in particular, is alkalinizing. It does contain antioxidant polyphenols that are anti-inflammatory. Most other authorities say that oils, in general, are, at best, neutral.

Alkaline or acid? There are a few foods that nobody can seem to agree on. Eggplant, artichoke, corn, mushrooms, and pineapple are so controversial that there is no consensus. And we can't just stick a piece of litmus paper in the food bowl because we know that some of these foods react differently after being digested. Use these in moderation, or check the pH of your body frequently and make adjustments.

Juices

Juicing removes the fiber from vegetables, so it can't make up your entire intake of these excellent foods. But it is a good way to concentrate the nutritive qualities of these alkalinizing foods. Besides, it's a lot easier to drink a glass of carrot juice than it is to eat the carrots it takes to make it! For a great source of alkaline mineral salts, drink your vegetables.

Green vegetable juice, in particular, is alkalinizing. Many authorities consider celery juice, rich in organic sodium, to be the most alkalinizing food you can consume. Watch out for large quantities of beet and carrot juices, which are especially sweet. While the whole versions of these vegetables are generally alkalinizing, the concentrated juices have high sugar contents.

Fruit juices, while good concentrated sources of nutrients and generally considered very detoxifying, are high in concentrated natural sugar and are thought to push pH to the acid side.

The pH Values of Selected Foods

Remember that we are concerned about how a food is metabolized: what it does to the body's pH when it is digested. The pH of a food may not always predict how that food will ultimately metabolize. A lemon, for example, is pretty acid in pH, but many authorities recommend eating lemons to alkalinize the body. The following list presents the pH values of selected foods:

Salt, 7.0
Watercress, 7.0
Cantaloupe, 7.0
Maple syrup, 6.7
Corn, 6.6
Black olives, canned, 6.6
Brussels sprouts, 6.5
Camembert cheese, 6.5
Endive, 6.5
Honey, 6.4
Brown rice syrup, 6.4

Dates, 6.3
Fish and shellfish, in general, 6.3
Soybeans, 6.3
Butter, 6.3
Cauliflower, 6.2
Lettuce, 6.2
Mushrooms, 6.2
Nuts and seeds, in general, 6.0
Grains (wheat, rice, barley, oat, rye, millet, quinoa, amaranth), 6.0
Espresso, 5.9

Peas, 5.9
White potatoes, 5.9
Celery, 5.9
Spinach, 5.8
Broccoli, 5.8
Parsley, 5.8
Garlic, 5.8
Avocado, 5.7
Cabbage, 5.7
Beef, 5.7
Persimmon, 5.6
Carrots, 5.6
Artichokes, 5.6
Cheese, in general, 5.6
Papaya, 5.5
Asparagus, 5.5
Onion, 5.5
Turnip greens, 5.5
Dried beans, in general, 5.5
White bread, 5.5
Radishes, 5.5
Turnips, 5.4
Sweet potatoes, 5.4
Parsnips, 5.3
Squash, 5.2
Parmesan cheese, 5.2
Molasses, 5.2
Pumpkin, 5.1
Walnuts, 5.0
Coffee, 5.0
Bell peppers, 4.9
Bananas, 4.8
Figs, 4.8
Cottage cheese, 4.7
Roquefort cheese, 4.7
String beans, 4.6

Tomatoes, 4.5
Guava, 4.5
Wine and beer, 4.5
Asian pears, 4.4
Eggplants, 4.3
Mangoes, 4.2
Pears, 4.1
Cherries, 4.0
Tomatilloes, 4.0
Yogurt, 4.0
Prune juice, 4.0
Raisins, 3.9
Peaches, 3.9
Mayonnaise, 3.9
Plums, 3.7
Apricots, 3.7
Apple juice, 3.6
Blackberries, 3.6
Strawberries, 3.6
Boysenberries, 3.6
Pineapple juice, 3.6
Grapefruits, 3.5
Oranges, 3.5
Orange juice, 3.5
Blueberries, 3.4
Sauerkraut, 3.4
Cucumbers, 3.4
Raspberries, 3.3
Dill pickles, 3.2
Grapefruit juice, 3.2
Rhubarb, 3.1
Cranberry juice, 2.7
Lemons, 2.3
Lemon juice, 2.0
Limes, 1.9

Substitutes for Acidic Foods

Cookies made with maple syrup? Soy milk on your cereal? Why not? Most Americans turn out to be too acidic. If you are like most folks, you will see a lot of the foods you eat on the acid side of Table 10.2. If you are working toward substituting these acid-producing foods with alkaline alternatives, take a look at the alkaline options and reflect on how you could switch to them, at least a bit more often. For most people, it works much better to go slow. Integrate a few changes, make them habits, and move on to the next challenge.

Sugar

All authorities in the field are unanimous in their condemnation of refined carbohydrates, especially white sugar. Refined carbohy-

Table 10.2. Alkaline Options for Acid Foods	
Acid Foods	**Alkaline Options**
Acid condiments (ketchup, mayonnaise, vinegar)	Garlic, herbs, kelp, lemon rind
Coffee	Herbal coffee substitutes (Postum, Roastaroma)
Cow's milk	Nut milk, rice milk, soy milk
Fried foods	Baked foods
Red meat (beef, lamb, pork, veal)	Tofu, veggie burgers
Salt	Salt substitute (Bragg's Aminos)
White bread	Bread made from other grains (amaranth, millet, oat, quinoa, brown rice, soy)
White sugar	Barley malt, brown rice syrup, honey, maple syrup, rice bran syrup

drates increase acidity and worsen the typical Western metabolic problem.

The average American eats over 20 percent more sugar (about 25 more pounds per person per year) than in 1986. According to the Center for Science in the Public Interest, the current estimate for the average American's consumption of caloric sweeteners (sugar, corn syrup, and the like) is around 152 pounds a year.

The excess calories make people fat. The sweeteners are "empty" calories: they contain no nutrients, and they take the dietary place of nutrient-rich whole foods. Refined sweeteners promote excess insulin release, increasing the risk for dysglycemia, diabetes, cardiovascular disease, and obesity. Dr. Lynn August asks, "What is the right amount of sugar and caloric sweeteners?" Her answer? "None."[5]

According to Dr. Gaby, eating sugar may also deplete our bodies of calcium. Numerous studies over the years have shown that a high-sugar diet causes urinary calcium to increase.[6,7] A recent French study showed that a single chocolate bar containing 55 grams of sucrose produced a striking increase in blood triglycerides and urine calcium.[8]

To make matters worse, when people with a history of calcium oxalate kidney stones, or their relatives, were given 100 grams of sugar, they excreted even more calcium. In the body, 99 percent of stored calcium is located in the bones, so the increase in calcium excretion caused by sugar probably means that it is leaching from bone. Therefore, this information suggests that a diet high in sugar may lower the calcium content of bone. This certainly backs up what Dr. Brown and Dr. Lark have to say about sugar and bone mass.

To add to our scientific information, a 1987 study investigated the idea that eating sugar, known to increase blood insulin, would inhibit the reabsorption of calcium through the kidney. In other words, the calcium would be excreted in the urine. You guessed it. That's just what happened. And it also happened to zinc and sodium, two other alkaline minerals.[9]

A significant study came out in *The American Journal of Clinical Nutrition* in 2002 that again gave support to this connection. In the Framingham Osteoporosis Study, scientists with the U.S. Department of Agriculture Human Nutrition Research Center on Aging at Tufts University in Boston studied 907 older Americans to determine the dietary factors connected with bone mineral density (BMD). They concluded, "High candy consumption was associated with low BMD in both men and women." In fact, candy consumption was the most substantial predictor of low BMD in the study.[10]

Scientists have suggested that refined sugar consumption is one of the factors that encourage kidney stones. It also looks like people with kidney stones, or with just a family history of kidney stones, are especially susceptible to the unfavorable effects of sugar. Dr. Gaby speculates that perhaps what people with kidney stones and those with osteoporosis have in common is an increased negative response to refined sugar.

And the bottom-line question really is: Does eating a lot of sugar cause diabetes? Time after time, studies have found little relationship between total carbohydrate intake and diabetes risk. Using total carbohydrate intake, however, does not take into account the blood sugar effect or insulin demand of various forms of carbohydrates.

A study in the *Journal of the American Medical Association* looked at this issue.[11] The report was part of a longitudinal study of diet and lifestyle factors in relation to chronic diseases (the Nurses Health Study) that involved more than 65,000 women, ages forty to sixty-five in 1986. All were free of cardiovascular disease, cancer, and diabetes at the beginning of the study. The subjects completed a detailed dietary questionnaire from which the scientists calculated the usual intake of dietary fiber, glycemic load, and dietary glycemic index. (Glycemic index is a ranking of foods based on the glucose response and insulin demand they produce for the carbohydrate they contain. The insulin output produced may vary among foods that contain the same amount of carbohydrate. Other factors also influence the absorption of any given food, and not all types of carbohydrates produce the same insulin response. On a scale of 100, white bread has a glycemic index of 100, while broccoli has an index of 45.) The patients were followed for six years to chart the number who developed diabetes.

Of the 65,000 women, more than 900 developed diabetes. The women eating foods with the highest glycemic indexes (the carbohydrates that provoked the highest insulin demands) had the highest incidence of diabetes. Consuming high-fiber whole grains reduced the chance of developing the disease. Cola beverages, white bread, white rice, and potatoes were risk factors. Cold breakfast cereal and yogurt were associated with prevention. The scientists concluded that diets with high refined carbohydrates and low fiber content led to a chronic high demand for insulin and increased the occurrence of diabetes, independent of other dietary factors and currently known risk factors. Their final advice is that grains should be consumed in minimally refined forms to reduce diabetes.

Excessive sugar may also contribute to cancer. Proponents of the pH diet theories, in their various forms, have consistently maintained that excess acidity ups cancer risk. Researchers from the University of Toronto completed a study in 2001 that found that glycemic index and glycemic load were associated with increased breast cancer risk.[12] High insulin and the condition of insulin resistance play a role in increased breast cancer.

Some carbohydrates increase glucose and insulin concentration to a greater degree than others. Insulin stimulates the production of growth factors, which are in turn connected with an increased incidence of breast cancer. At centers in Canada, Italy, and France, investigators evaluated interviews with 2,569 women with confirmed breast cancer and 2,588 controls. Based on a food questionnaire, the authors calculated the patients' average daily glycemic index and glycemic load. The higher the glycemic content of the food, the greater was the occurrence of breast cancer. Consumption of foods with a high glycemic index, such as white bread, increased breast cancer risk the most. Menopausal status, alcohol consumption, and physical activity did not affect the relationship between dietary glycemic content and breast cancer risk. The scientists concluded that, based on this data, the glycemic response of the total diet has a moderate and direct association with breast cancer risk and that the resulting high insulin and insulin resistance might contribute to breast cancer development.

Honey, in contrast to white sugar, according to Dr. Dipasquale, has long been considered one of the best pH balancers. In fact, honey is the least acidic sweetener on the scale developed by Dr. Young. When used, as often recommended, with apple cider vinegar, which Dr. Brown says is converted to a weak base, this combination helps balance body pH.

Other whole sweeteners—maple syrup, molasses, barley malt syrup, and rice bran syrup—are considered to be far less acid producing because they contain less total sugar and they come with an assortment of alkalinizing minerals built in. But there is a limit. Ultimately, all carbohydrates break down into acids. Be moderate in your use of sweeteners; they really are just treats and not necessary on a daily basis.

For several years, I was the director of the nutritional therapy department of 3HO Superhealth, a holistic hospital in Tucson, Arizona. This hospital was accredited by the Joint Commission on Accreditation of

Hospitals and was the first natural healing hospital to be covered by conventional insurance providers, including Blue Cross and military insurance. When I worked at the hospital, I got to see the true compelling attraction of white sugar. I think it is the most addictive (if we can use that term for this chemical) substance in America. Most of the hospital's patients were with us for drug rehabilitation and would stay for six weeks or so, until they had become stabilized and had the opportunity to put together a drugless life to which to return in the world.

Every patient was with us for at least one drug of choice—the one that ultimately pulled them down and helped them hit rock bottom. But they were *always* addicted to several substances. Most of them smoked. Most of them drank to excess. Almost all drank coffee by the gallon. And every single one of them was a sugar junkie. So, from the moment they walked through the door, they were kicking their hard drugs of choice as well as caffeine, nicotine, and sugar. We got very good at helping people through multidrug withdrawal.

Of course, we were a natural healing hospital, so we did not serve sugar anywhere on the hospital campus. We also did not serve coffee, allow smoking, and of course, tolerated no illegal drugs. We even minimized legal drugs given under a doctor's care.

When patients missed bed check and I had to go on patrol to reel them in, did I go to the street to find them scoring dope? No way. There was a doughnut shop down the road. I knew I could drive right there and wrangle 'em back to the corral.

Longtime heroin users told us that heroin withdrawal was easy compared to sugar withdrawal. After all, they had been sugar addicts since infancy.

I would often be chatting with a patient who was close to being discharged after spending a transformative forty days at the hospital. When we talked about relapse possibilities, the feeling was often the same. Did patients lie in bed fantasizing about a shot of heroin? Nope; their dreams were filled with cadres of dancing pastries.

Protein

According to Dr. Gaby, the American diet tends to contain too much protein. He claims that studies have indicated that excessive protein in the diet may encourage bone loss. When you eat more protein, the urinary excretion of calcium rises. The digestion of protein liberates acidic breakdown products. As we know, calcium is mobilized to buffer these chemicals. Dr. Gaby maintains that science has shown that people who eat a vegetarian diet have stronger bones later in life than those who eat meat.

The amino acid methionine, which is abundant in animal protein, is converted in the body to homocysteine. It now looks as if this chemical, which has become known as a cardiovascular disease risk factor marker, is capable of causing bone loss.

Animal flesh contains phosphorus, a necessary nutrient. But Dr. Gaby says that excessive consumption contributes to osteoporosis. One of the breakdown products, phosphoric acid, must be buffered by calcium. This probably explains in part why excessive protein has an adverse effect on bone.

Grains

All carbohydrates eventually break down into blood sugar (glucose), the moment-to-moment fuel for our cells. As this glucose is oxidized by the cells for fuel, to provide body heat, acids are produced. That's just the fact. So all grains eventually contribute to the acid load, regardless of the form in which they are consumed. Of course, so do the other macronutrients. Since we require the macronutrients to sustain life, however, we can't go without them. It's just that we don't want to overdo any one foodstuff, and we want to complement these acid-forming macronutrients with alkaline foods.

Refined grains, seeds from which the bran and germ have been removed, are the "white" versions—white flour, white rice. These are digested rapidly and are speedily metabolized into glucose. This rapid assimilation creates a spike of acid with which the body may have trouble dealing. Out come the alkalinizing minerals from the skeleton. Unfortunately, just like with your checkbook, it might be easier for the body to make a withdrawal from the mineral bank account than it will be for it to cover the withdrawal with a deposit a while later. Oops—overdrawn!

During the past century, people began to eat large amounts of refined grains, such as white bread instead of whole wheat bread, and white rice instead of brown rice.

Eating whole grains has many advantages. With the bran and germ still intact, all the original fiber remains in the grain. In addition to all the dietary benefits of the fiber, it also slows down digestion of the starch, retarding the acid spike. The whole grain contains almost all of the other nutrients in the grain: the alkalinizing minerals, especially magnesium; the vitamins; and the essential fatty acids. Dr. Dipasquale says that "brown rice is more alkaline than white rice, because the bran and germ have been preserved."

Besides, whole grains in the diet may reduce the risk of diabetes and cardiovascular disease. Research from the Framingham Offspring Study shows that upping the intake of whole grain foods may hold back type 2 diabetes and cardiovascular disease. Previous epidemiological research has indicated that diets rich in whole grains (dark bread, popcorn, oatmeal, brown rice) may ward off these conditions, even though we don't understand much about how whole grains provide their protective effects. The average whole grain consumption in the United States is only one serving per day, in spite of the dietary guidelines that recommend eating several. Almost all grain products devoured in the United States are refined.

A study of 2,941 subjects in the *American Journal of Clinical Nutrition* found that people who ate more whole grains had better body fat readings, low-density lipoprotein (LDL) cholesterol, and fasting insulin. The researchers concluded that the benefits were mainly connected with the magnesium and fiber contents of the whole grains.[13,14]

Wheat, in particular, is problematic. To begin with, it has a higher protein content than most grains. Dr. Lark and Dr. Dipasquale say it is acid forming and recommend that you substitute other grains that have less impact on acidity. Wheat is widely thought to be one of the top three allergy-producing foods for Americans. Dr. Dipsaquale feels that millet and buckwheat are less acid forming than wheat.

The recent trend toward applauding carbohydrates, as demonstrated in the current food pyramid, has led to misinterpretation. The benefits come largely from unrefined grains. Many people, however, in trying to emulate this diet, miss the distinction and load up on refined grains, which are much more problematic.

Recently, the high-carbohydrate diet has come under fire from a cadre of experts. Again, the statistics in Americans are based on the recent practice of concentrating on white flour products. A study of 5,000 Italian women published in *The Lancet* indicates that starch, not fat, was linked to an increase in breast cancer. The scientists could not decisively explain their results, but consider that a preponderance of wheat starch could be harmful. Liberal amounts of olive oil had a protective effect.[15]

Salt

Frankly, authorities differ a bit about salt. Pure table salt is composed of sodium and chlorine. Sodium is alkalinizing. Chlorine is acidifying. Salt actually has a neutral pH of 7.0 when dissolved in water.[16] Most authorities, including Dr. Lark, put salt in the acid category.

Products called sea salt may not be much different. Just because salt comes from the sea does not necessarily mean that it has any other significant mineral content. One popular health food brand, for instance, is 99.99 percent sodium chloride, .005 percent calcium sulfate, .003 percent magnesium chloride, and .002 percent sodium sulfate.[17] (Federal standards require that all table salt products be at least 97.5 percent sodium chloride, so there's not a lot of room for much else.) Unprocessed salt may have a somewhat higher trace mineral content. (One popular brand of unprocessed sea salt has 1.8 percent trace elements—pretty skimpy.)[18]

Natural sea salt contains a host of additional minerals, most of them alkalinizing. It just might not have much. On the whole, Dr. Brown says that natural sea salt is alkaline forming.

Dr. August recommends that you drink water according to your thirst and eat salt according to your taste. She claims that if you do not crave salt or if you have an aversion to it, you are salt deficient. The same is true of water. She suggests that you start by eating a little more salt than you do now. Increase the daily amount a little at a time, without using so much that it ruins the taste of your food. If you keep increasing your salt intake, you will eventually develop a desire for salt.[19]

If salt makes you retain water, she maintains that you are probably eating too many carbohydrates or not enough protein.

On the other hand, macrobiotic proponents often recommend salt as an alternative to the excess sweetness of the North American diet. Dr. Michael Tierra says that George Ohsawa knew that the Western mind was not prepared to understand the dynamic nature of yin and yang theory and would have difficulty understanding the important TCM concept of yin deficiency. Dr. Tierra says, "So from [Ohsawa's] perspective salt was important because it increased one's capacity to retain fluid which in turn would help the body to retain warmth."

In a recent challenge to medical dogma, a Canadian researcher from Toronto's Mt. Sinai Hospital, Dr. Alexander Logan, reviewed fifty-six studies and decided that, surprisingly, sodium intake has no noteworthy effect on blood pressure. Instead, he found a number of negative effects from restricting salt intake, including disturbances in cholesterol and calcium metabolism.[20]

According to Dr. August, table salt is anabolic; it increases body size.

Phosphorus

Phosphorus is often regarded as a twin nutrient to calcium. It is a major mineral. The average body contains about 1.5 pounds of it. This important mineral is involved, directly or indirectly, in nearly every cellular function. Alongside calcium, phosphorus builds and hardens bones and teeth. In bone tissue, the calcium to phosphorus ratio is two to one. Phosphorus plays an important role in transforming proteins, fats, and carbohydrates into fuel. It makes fats water soluble, assisting them in entering the bloodstream; strengthens cell walls; and transports nutrients and hormones throughout the body.

Phosphorus is an important mineral for constructing bone tissue, but it shifts pH to the acid side. For most modern Americans, that is a problem. Phosphorus in the diet creates phosphoric acid in the body. In fact, cola beverages contain straight phosphoric acid to give them that "snappy" taste. Phosphoric acid, in any form, adds to the acid load and must be buffered by the alkaline mineral reservoir.

Active teenage girls who drink cola drinks are five times more likely to have bone fractures than girls who don't consume soda, according to a study of 460 ninth- and tenth-grade girls. A Harvard researcher found that any type of carbonated drink increased the chance of having a bone fracture. Who had the greatest increases? The girls who drank cola beverages and reported their physical activity as either high-level or vigorous.[21] Two similar earlier studies by the same researcher had found strong correlations between carbonated beverages and bone fractures in active females.

Another similar study, this time in rats and done in Mexico, showed the same result: Cola drinks, containing phosphoric acid, reduced bone mineral density.[22]

Most Americans already eat plenty of phosphorus, as the mineral is abundant in animal flesh. The likelihood is that you have more than enough in your body already and do not need to add more from colas.

In Dr. Gaby's opinion, "High-phosphorus beverages such as colas (which also contain a lot of sugar and caffeine) are among the worst foods imaginable for someone trying to prevent osteoporosis."

Potassium

A team of researchers led by Anthony Sebastian, from the Department of Medicine and the General Clinic Research Center at the University of California, San Francisco, recently reported on an investigation that disclosed that the typical Western diet generates slight chronic systemic metabolic acidosis in humans. According to the scientists, such a diet accelerates aging, degrades muscle and bone, and suppresses growth hormone secretion. Alkaline diets have the opposite effects.

The idea is that humans should be better adapted physiologically to the diet with which our ancestors evolved, compared to the diet we have been eating since the agricultural revolution, which was a mere 10,000 years ago. Industrialization was only 200 years ago, and it radically adjusted dietary patterns.

The mismatch between our genetically determined nutritional requirements and our current diet has created many health problems. The scientists reasoned that some of these problems might be a consequence of the deficiency of alkaline potassium salts. These salts were amply present in the plant foods that our ancestors ate in abundance. The contemporary diet has exchanged those salts for copious sodium chloride, which was meager in the potassium-rich plant foods of the past. Deficiency of potassium in the diet increases the net systemic load, say the scientists. They point out that clinically recognized chronic metabolic acidosis has negative effects on the body, including growth retardation in children, decrease in muscle and bone mass in adults, and kidney stone formation.

The researchers wondered if a lifetime of eating diets that deliver excess loads of acid to the body contributes to the decrease in bone and muscle mass and growth hormone secretion that we have become accustomed to regarding as normal parts of aging. Are modern humans suffering from chronic, diet-induced low-grade systemic metabolic acidosis?

It has previously been shown that the current net acid-producing diets do indeed typically cause low-grade systemic metabolic acidosis and that the severity of the acidosis increases with age, in relation to the normally occurring age-related decline in kidney function. They determined that offsetting the diet net acid load with supplements of potassium bicarbonate improved calcium and phosphorus balance, nitrogen balance, and decline in growth hormone secretion. Furthermore, it reduced bone resorption rates. They did all this without restricting dietary salt.

Earlier studies had estimated the dietary acid load from the amount of animal protein in the diet. Remember that protein metabolism yields sulfuric acid as an end product. Cross-cultural epidemiologic studies have found that hip fracture incidence in older women was related to animal protein intake, caused by the acid load from protein. They found that plant food intake tended to be protective against hip fracture. Countries that ate more plants and less meat had less hip fracture. In a more homogeneous population of white elderly women residents of the United States, the same pattern was observed. These eminent scientists argue that any level of acidosis may be unacceptable, based on how our bodies have evolved, and that a low-grade metabolic alkalosis may be the optimal state for humans.[23]

Vegetables, as a whole, are very rich in potassium. Upping your vegetable consumption to Dr. Brown's recommended two servings with lunch and two with dinner will easily fulfill your quota of this main alkalinizing nutrient.

Bernard Jensen, D.C., a pioneer in the study of pH, claimed that sundried Italian olives, cured in sea salt, are the highest potassium-containing foods. He suggested preparing them by soaking ten olives in 2 cups of hot water. Dr. Jensen also maintained that potato *peels* make a great potassium food.[24] Peel potatoes thick and simmer the peels. Add other alkalinizing vegetables, such as celery, for flavor, if you wish. Dr. Jensen used this formula for arthritis. I can say that I have used this recipe for thirty years with patients having arthritis and have had very positive responses.

Celery is widely considered to be the most cooling and alkalinizing food available. Dr. Jensen specifically recommended it many times. Yogi Bhajan has hailed its virtues for years. Celery is very rich in alkaline organic sodium (not sodium chloride). It is powerfully anti-inflammatory and relaxing.

Since celery is very fibrous, it is hard to chomp down very much at a sitting. Steam it or, better yet, juice it. At 3HO Superhealth, celery juice was one of our main treatments for anxiety and insomnia. About 8 to 16 ounces will put you right to sleep. It is so cooling that a 10-ounce glass will abort a hay fever attack. Dr. Jensen combined prune juice with, believe it or not, celery juice to nourish the nervous system.

So What Can We Do?

Overall, it's balance that counts. If you apply the principles we have been discussing, you will bring your metabolism into line. The more disciplined you are, the faster it will happen. For best success, focus on the big factors: Reduce the worst offenders in your diet, and up the quantity of the foods that will balance the pH.

Start with a basic program to alkalinize your body with diet. Reduce red meat, sugar, refined flour, and excessive amounts of sweet fruits. Increase vegetables, especially green ones. Add in fruits, especially low-sugar varieties. Replace cola drinks and other unhealthy beverages with water and vegetable juices. As you begin to change your diet in these general ways, you will find your pH measurements beginning to shift. You're on your way!

Alkalinizing Recipes

Alkalinizing food can be healthy, but can it taste decent? What about all those bitter vegetables and chewy, pasty grains? And no éclairs? Since most folks will need to head in the alkaline direction, it *will* mean upping the vegetables and grains in the diet, but we can do it deliciously. Here are some great examples of healthy foods that might just change your mind about health food.

In all the years I've been around people who were working on their health, the single most important imperative I've learned is to go at your own pace when you make changes. If you're a plodder, plod. I've seen many folks, with all the best intentions, go home and empty their cupboards. After filling them back up with healthy food, they stand back and admire their accomplishment. But then comes dinnertime. Unfortunately, the new regime didn't come with cooking lessons. A week later, guess what's sneaked back in to fill up the cupboard again. The same things that had been thrown in the garbage just a week earlier.

Total, sweeping change does not work for most people. Instead, start with one change that you can accomplish that will motivate you. When you've mastered that one, and it's a habit, snap off another challenge. In a few months or a year, your cupboard will be full of healthy food, and it won't be just trophy foods. You will actually be eating and enjoying it.

To help get you started on your road to balance, following are some recipes for healthy, alkalinizing foods.

Vegetable Dishes

ALKALINE CASSEROLE

2 medium eggplants, cubed
2 medium potatoes, cubed
2 medium green peppers, seeded and cubed
2 medium onions, peeled and cubed
2 medium zucchini or other mild squash, cubed
1 medium tomato, seeded and cubed
¼ pound green beans, cut into pieces
¼ pound mushrooms, any variety, chopped
3 cloves garlic, chopped
2 teaspoons dill weed or tarragon, crushed
2 teaspoons oregano, crushed
2 teaspoons basil, crushed
Salt and pepper to taste
4 ounces vegetable broth
2 tablespoons olive oil

Soak eggplant cubes in salted water for 2 hours. Preheat oven to 375°. Drain eggplant and place in a large mixing bowl. Add remaining vegetables and stir to combine. Add seasonings, broth, and oil, and stir again. Place in a casserole dish and bake at 375° for 2 to 3 hours, until vegetables are thoroughly cooked. For moister consistency, cover casserole dish during baking.

Yield: 8 servings

BEET-CARROT CASSEROLE

1 bunch beets
1 pound carrots
2 bunches scallions, chopped
3 cloves garlic, minced
Ghee or vegetable oil
Soy sauce
Ground black pepper
1 pound grated cheese

Scrub beets and carrots. Steam beets whole (don't cut off roots or stems). After about 15 to 20 minutes, add carrots. Steam until tender but firm. Then remove outer peels from beets and carrots. (These should easily slip off.) Grate using a coarse grater. Keep beets and carrots separate to preserve their distinct colors. Sauté scallions and garlic in oil or ghee until tender. Toss with beets, carrots, and black pepper. Place in a casserole dish. Sprinkle with soy sauce. If desired, cover with grated cheese and broil until cheese is melted and golden.

Comment: The cheese in this recipe is only a compensation for American tastes. Feel free to omit or adjust cheese, based on pH needs of the individual. According to Ayurveda, this dish is cleansing to the liver and digestive tract. For cleansing, eat only this dish for one week in the spring or fall.

Yield: 4 to 6 servings

From *Foods for Health and Healing* by Yogi Bhajan (Pamona, CA: Arcline Publications, 1989) copyright © 1969–2002 by Yogi Bhajan. Used with permission.

FENNEL AND GREENS SALAD

Mixed salad greens or spinach leaves, washed and
torn into bite-sized pieces
Fresh fennel bulbs, sliced

Ginger Salad Dressing

¼ cup vegetable oil
2 tablespoons plain or toasted sesame oil
2 tablespoons rice or other vinegar or lemon juice
2 tablespoons soy sauce
1 tablespoon honey (optional)
1 to 3 green onions and/or garlic cloves, chopped
1 tablespoon fresh ginger, minced

Place the greens in a large bowl and set aside. In a separate bowl, combine the dressing ingredients and stir until well blended. Pour dressing over greens and toss to coat.

Yield: 1 cup dressing

FENNEL SALSA

1 fresh fennel bulb, diced
10 green olives, pitted and diced
½ cup chopped orange sections
1 tablespoon orange juice
Lemon juice, to taste
Salt and pepper, to taste

In a large bowl, combine the fennel, olives, and orange. Add the juices, salt, and pepper, and mix well.

Yield: 3 cups

GREEN BEANS WITH ALLSPICE

1 tablespoon vegetable oil
2 to 4 cloves garlic, minced
1 pound fresh green beans, washed and trimmed,
    left whole or cut to any size
2 teaspoons ground allspice
Salt and pepper, or herb mixture, to taste

In a medium saucepan, heat the oil over low heat. Add the garlic and cook, stirring, until lightly browned. Add the green beans and sauté briefly. Add just enough water to steam the beans. Bring to a boil and stir in the seasonings. Cover and simmer briefly, until the beans are cooked through but still crunchy.

Yield: 4 servings

Rice and Bean Dishes

BALANCING METALS AND VITAMINS

Rice, to taste
Onions, to taste
Chopped orange peel (include white strings inside), to taste
Cooked chickpeas, to taste
Red chiles, to taste
Green vegetables, to taste
Sesame oil, to taste
Ginseng, to taste (optional)

Boil rice, add onions, cook until soft. Add orange peel and chickpeas. Add red chiles to taste. Add green vegetables and oil to taste. If desired, add ginseng to taste.

From *The Ancient Art of Self-Healing* by Amir Arberman (Royal Oak, MI: Arbor Press, 2001) copyright © 1969–2002 by Yogi Bhajan. Used with permission.

BARLEY BEAN PILAF

1 teaspoon olive oil
1 cup diced onion
2 cloves garlic, minced
½ cup diced celery
3 cups diced fresh mushrooms, any variety
3 cups water
½ cup dry barley
2 cups cooked white beans
3 teaspoons soy sauce

In a large saucepan, heat the oil over low heat. Add the onion and garlic, and sauté until lightly browned. Add the celery and continue sautéing until the celery starts to become transparent. Add the mushrooms and continue sautéing until soft and thoroughly cooked. Add the water and soy sauce, and bring the mixture to a boil. Add the barley, cover, and simmer until the barley is fully cooked. Add the beans and continue simmering until the mixture reaches a stewlike consistency.

Yield: 8 servings

MUNG BEANS AND RICE

1 cup mung beans
1 cup basmati rice
9 cups water
4 to 6 cups chopped assorted vegetables (carrot, celery, zucchini, broccoli, etc.)
2 onions, chopped
⅓ cup minced ginger root
8 to 10 cloves garlic, minced
1 heaping teaspoon turmeric
½ teaspoon black pepper
1 heaping teaspoon garam masala (curry powder)
1 teaspoon crushed red chiles (to taste)
1 tablespoon basil
2 bay leaves
Seeds of 5 cardamom pods
Salt or soy sauce to taste

Wash beans and rice. Bring water to boil, add beans, and let boil over medium-high flame for about 45 minutes. Prepare vegetables. Add vegetables and rice to cooking beans. Heat oil (about ½ cup) in large frying pan. Add onion, ginger and garlic. Sauté over medium-high flame until browned. Add spices (not salt or herbs). When nicely well done, combine onion mixture with cooking beans and rice. Stir often to prevent scorching. Add herbs. Continue cooking until totally and completely well done, over a medium-high flame, stirring often. The consistency should be rich, thick, and soupy, with ingredients mixed. Serve with yogurt, or with cheese melted over the top. Prepare less spicy for elderly or small children.

Comment: Other varieties of rice may be substituted. Cook brown rice very well.

Yield: 6 to 8 servings

PARSLEY PILAF

2 onions, chopped
½ cup ghee
2 teaspoons ajwain seed
1 teaspoon ground red pepper (or more to taste)
1 tablespoon turmeric
1 teaspoon black pepper
2 crushed bay leaves
1 cup basmati rice
2 cups chopped potato (skins on)
1 cup parsley

Sauté onions in ghee. Add spices. Cook until browned. Add rice, potato, and parsley. Stir for a while. Add water (to steam rice), cover, and cook for another 15 minutes. Serve with yogurt for extra stamina.

Comment: This recipe is considered to be particularly good for men. Of course, women can eat it as well. Parsley is diuretic, and Ayurveda says it has the effect of reducing stress on the prostate gland by reducing water retention in the pelvis. Other varieties of rice may be substituted. Cook brown rice very well.

According to Ayurveda, this recipe is detoxifying and diuretic. It is regarded as a brain food that treats headache, head heaviness, and drowsiness. You can eat it as a mono diet for a few days or a week or two for medicinal value.

Yield: 4 to 6 servings

TRINITY RICE

1 cup basmati rice
½ to ¾ cup ghee
2 onions, chopped
2 cloves garlic, peeled and sliced
1-inch ginger root, peeled and grated
1 tomato, peeled
4 to 5 cups assorted chopped vegetables

Rinse basmati rice thoroughly. Sauté spices in ghee until golden brown. Add onion, garlic, and ginger ("trinity roots") and stir slowly until onions begin falling apart. Then add tomato, assorted vegetables, and rice, along with 4 cups of water. Cover and let simmer on a low heat, checking frequently. Add water as necessary. Cook until vegetables are soft and rice is done.

Comment: Ayurveda recommends this dish especially for convalescence. It builds stamina and is used in a training diet for athletes. Other varieties of rice may be substituted. Cook brown rice very well.

Yield: 4 servings

From *The Ancient Art of Self-Healing* by Amir Arberman (Royal Oak, MI: Arbor Press, 2001) copyright © 1969–2002 by Yogi Bhajan. Used with permission.

Main Dishes

JALAPEÑO PANCAKES

Equal parts finely chopped ginger and cauliflower
1 finely chopped jalapeño pepper per pancake
Ajwain seeds
Crushed red chiles
Black pepper
Bragg's Aminos or soy sauce
Equal parts bran and whole wheat flour
    (approximately ½ cup each per pancake)
Enough water to make a thick batter

Mix all ingredients, using spices, ginger, and cauliflower to tolerance. Cook on griddle with nonstick substance (lecithin, etc.—batter is very sticky). Cook on *low* heat for about ½ hour (15 minutes per side). Dose is usually two large pancakes per day—one in the A.M. and one in the P.M. with one glass of skim milk.

Comment: Bragg's Aminos is a soy sauce substitute. To purchase, see the Resource List, page 285.

Yield: 1 pancake for every ½ cup of flour

From *The Ancient Art of Self-Healing* by Amir Arberman (Royal Oak, MI: Arbor Press, 2001) copyright © 1969–2002 by Yogi Bhajan. Used with permission.

SWEET BEAN ROLLUPS

3 teaspoons vegetable oil
1 onion, minced
4 cloves garlic, minced
6 cups cooked kidney beans, mashed
4 cups cooked sweet potatoes, mashed
3 tablespoons soy sauce
2 teaspoons cumin powder
2 teaspoons oregano
Cayenne, to taste
12 large whole wheat or wheat-free chapattis, steamed
Cheese, shredded (optional)

Preheat oven to 350°. In a medium skillet or saucepan, heat the oil. Add the onion and garlic, and sauté until lightly browned. In a large pan, combine the mashed beans, mashed sweet potatoes, sautéed onion and garlic, and seasonings. If necessary, add water to achieve appropriate consistency for rollup filling. Divide filling among warm chapattis. Add cheese, if desired, and roll up. Place in baking dish and bake for 12 minutes.

Yield: 12 rollups

Soups

DONG QUAI SOUP

2 tablespoons vegetable oil
4 ½ cups chopped vegetables (carrot, onion, cabbage, etc.)
1 block tofu
1 cup chopped mushrooms
1 ounce dong quai root, sliced
5 cups water
2 tablespoons miso
3 to 10 cloves garlic, chopped
Spices (salt, pepper, tamari, ginger, etc.), to taste

In a large soup pot, heat the oil. Add the chopped vegetables and sauté until cooked. Add the remaining ingredients and bring to a boil. Reduce the heat and simmer for 1 hour or more, until the garlic is soft. Remove the dong quai slices before serving.

Yield: 8 servings

MINERAL BROTH

5 cups celery and/or celery tops, coarsely chopped
4 cups carrot and/or beet tops (can include roots), coarsely chopped
2 cups ½-inch-thick potato peels, coarsely chopped
Coarsely chopped onion, to taste
Coarsely chopped garlic cloves, to taste
½ teaspoon herbal seasoning
2 quarts water

In a large soup pot, bring all the ingredients to a boil over medium heat. Reduce the heat and simmer for about 20 minutes. Strain and serve the broth as a drink or use as a soup base.

Yield: 3 quarts

NETTLE SOUP

1 ½ quarts water
2 quarts nettle leaves, rinsed
1 to 2 ounces chopped scallions, onion, and/or garlic
2 tablespoons butter or oil
3 tablespoons flour
Vegetable broth, to taste
Seasonings, to taste

In a large soup pot, heat water to boiling. Add nettle leaves, reduce heat, and simmer until tender. Remove from heat and strain, reserving liquid. Place nettle leaves in blender, add scallions, onion, and/or garlic, and process. In large saucepan, melt butter over low heat. Add flour and cook, stirring, into a roux. Add nettle water, continuing to stir. Add blended nettle mixture and seasonings, and continue to simmer until well cooked.

Comment: Collect nettles in the early spring, when the leaves are about an inch long. Wear gloves whenever handling nettles.

Yield: 10 servings

Beverages

GREEN BLENDER DRINK

Any combination of green vegetables (sprouts, green peppers, green beans, broccoli, spinach, celery, etc.), coarsely chopped
Water

Place vegetables in a blender or food processor, filling compartment to the top, then add water to cover. Blend until completely liquefied, strain, and pour into glasses.

Comment: This is a quick way to tank up on alkalinizing vegetables without a juicer.

Yield: 4 servings

YOGI TEA

This is the original recipe given by Yogi Bhajan.

For each 8-ounce cup, start with 10 ounces of water. For convenience, make at least 4 cups of tea at one time.

For each cup of boiling water, add:

> 3 whole cloves
> 4 whole green cardamom pods
> 4 whole black peppercorns
> ½ stick cinnamon
> 1 slice of fresh ginger root (optional)

Boil for 20 to 30 minutes, then add ¼ teaspoon any black or green tea. Let sit for 1 or 2 minutes and then add ½ cup milk and reheat. Strain and serve with honey to taste.

Comment: Black pepper is a blood purifier, cardamom is for the colon (gas), cloves are for the nervous system, and cinnamon is for the bones. Ginger has a delicious taste and is helpful when suffering from a cold, recovering from the flu, or for general physical weakness. The milk aids in the easy assimilation of the spices and avoids irritation to the colon. The black or green tea acts as an alloy for all of the ingredients, achieving a new chemical structure that makes the tea a healthful and delicious drink.

11

Body Balance in the Digestive Tract

Something must not be going so right with the American digestive system. I don't think that would be any surprise to anyone. A recent study found that members of 69 percent of households suffered one or more gastrointestinal symptoms during a three-month period.[1] A total of 44 percent experienced a problem with the bowel.

As you would expect, those having a functional gastrointestinal disorder have an increased rate of work or school absenteeism and physician visits. Furthermore, people with certain more painful gastrointestinal disorders, such as chronic abdominal pain, biliary pain, functional dyspepsia, or irritable bowel syndrome, have the highest absenteeism rates.

The Gastrointestinal Tract

Twisting its way to link your mouth and your rectum, your digestive tract is a fifteen-foot-long tube with a pretty simple job. Food goes in one end, gets chomped up, and is then demolished by acid, enzymes, and bacteria. Finally, the nutrients are absorbed into the bloodstream. The remnants are eliminated at the far end, in the large intestine.

The gastrointestinal tract is composed of four distinct parts: the esophagus, stomach, small intestine, and large intestine. Separated from each other by special muscles called sphincters, which normally stay tightly closed and which regulate the movement of food and food residues from one part to another, each section has its own job to do and corresponding herbal remedies.

Most food molecules can't be absorbed in the form in which they occur in foods, so one of the primary functions of the digestive system is to break apart food molecules, convert them to an absorbable form, and absorb the nutrients. This complex process takes place mainly in the mucous membranes of the digestive tube.

The digestive tract is a war zone, with the most intense fluids in the entire body blasting in to digest whatever stands in their path. The war is between nutrients, which the body tries to absorb, and toxins, which the body tries to kick out. The wonderfully multipurpose mucous membrane is a combination of physical barrier, fluid producer, and active immune organ.

Herbalists are as interested in what comes out of the human body as what goes into it. If food isn't properly digested or the waste products properly eliminated, it hardly matters what you put in your mouth.

Taming the Wily Bowel

Proper bowel timing includes the key concepts of transit time and regularity. The time it takes for a meal to go in the mouth and come out from the other end is referred to as "transit time." For a person who eats a healthy diet, free of refined, processed foods, thirty hours is an average transit time. Ayurveda says the ideal transit time is from eighteen to twenty-four hours. In our constipation-prone society, forty-eight hours, or even considerably more, is commonplace.

The hitch with lengthy transit time is that the longer the end products of digestion stay in our system, the more chance they have of decomposing into unhealthy compounds. And if bowel transit time is slow, increasing the time that fecal matter spends within the colon leads to greater absorption of water from the feces. More water is absorbed, resulting in harder, smaller stools that have more difficulty moving forward. Increasingly, evidence implicates slow transit constipation in the development of gallstones.[2]

Measure your transit time by swallowing something that colors the stool. Mark the time that you see the color in the feces. Charcoal powder, beets, and chlorophyll all work well.

Regularity is the interval between bowel movements. Depending on whom you ask, the gamut of recommendations runs from "two or three bowel movements a week is plenty" to "a bowel movement every day is essential." Mammals are designed so that each meal stimulates fecal movement and initiates a bowel movement. Most natural healing practitioners insist on at least one bowel movement per day or up to one per meal.

Mouth

This is where it all starts. The balance of pH begins in the mouth. Your teeth chop up food, mixing it with saliva. The slightly acid saliva begins to process food the moment it comes into contact with it. Valuable calcium salts, dissolved in the acid saliva, remineralize the teeth. Even fat and starch digestion begin in the mouth, with the enzymes lingual lipase, salivary amylase, and ptyalin.

Stomach

The stomach churns food through muscular action. In the swirling mass, fats are emulsified. About 1 to 2 liters of gastric juices are produced per day. These highly acidic juices mix the food mass with mucus, forming a ball of semidigested material called *chyme*.

The gastric juices include hydrochloric acid, which is secreted by the parietal cells, and pepsin, an enzyme that renders some minerals (especially calcium and iron) more absorbable. Gastric lipase begins making fats more water-soluble. The acid environment begins to break apart proteins into smaller units, called polypeptides, which in turn are made up of strings of amino acids. Stomach acid kills invading bacteria, producing a fundamentally sterile environment. This high-acid juice measures somewhere between pH 1.0 and 3.5, with the average normal fasting stomach pH between 1.0 and 2.0 (a million times more acidic than water).

Contractions move the food contents slowly toward the large intestine, normally requiring about an hour and a half to two hours for the first part of a meal to reach the large intestine, although the last portion of the meal may not make it there for five hours.

As folks age, the ability of the stomach to sustain the high acid output begins to decline, a condition known as hypochlorhydria. Dr. Roberta Lee claims that stomach acid can often be reduced by 40 percent by the time of menopause. She recommends a test of stomach acidity for her patients at risk for mineral malabsorption.

Chanchal Cabrera says that in the British herbal tradition, calamus root is thought to be an acid balancer. A dose of up to 5 milliliters of tincture per day will reduce acid, while higher doses stimulate acid production. In any case, Asian medicine has long used calamus as a digestive aid.

Michael T. Murray. N.D., a prominent naturopathic physician based in Seattle, says that if the stomach becomes too alkaline and the pH rises above 3.5, pepsin, the primary enzyme in the stomach involved in digesting protein, is inactivated.[3] If you use antacids to treat indigestion, you could undermine your body's ability to completely digest the protein you eat.

As above, so below—this is certainly true in digestion. As you can imagine, this low acid at the very top of the digestive tube wreaks havoc all the way down. When food is not properly broken down in the stomach, the body has difficulty completing the process throughout the tube.

The traditional medical view has been that overproduction of acid is a common problem, so most conventional medicines aim to lessen stomach acid. If this is the case, that therapy is appropriate. Both conditions—hyperchlorhydria and hypochlorhydria—can impair proper digestion. Ironically, they produce similar symptoms, including heartburn and indigestion. A Heidelberg gastrogram can accurately measure stomach pH so that therapy can be properly targeted.

Small Intestine

The small intestine is where the real action happens. Most of digestion and absorption occurs in the small intestine.

First, the pancreas secretes alkaline digestive juices, including bicarbonate, at a rate of about 2.5 liters per day, to neutralize food. In the pancreas secretions, the proteases trypsin, chymotrypsin, and carboxypeptidase digest proteins down further to oligopeptides and amino acids. Pancreatic amylase splits starch to maltose and lipase, and hydrolyzes diglycerides and triglycerides, creating long-chain fatty acids.

Then the liver enters the picture. The liver secretes about 700 milliliters of bile per day.

Gallbladder

The gallbladder, or "gall bladder," is a small pear-shaped sac located on the underside of the liver, in the upper right side of the abdomen. This pouch averages three to six inches in length and serves as a reservoir for bile, which is produced by the liver to help the body digest fatty foods. It is connected to the liver and small intestine by small tubes called bile ducts.

Bile is a watery, greenish yellow fluid produced by the liver that aids in the digestion of fatty foods and assists in the absorption of certain vitamins and minerals. It contains water, bile salts (substances that break up fat), bile pigments (such as *bilirubin*, the pigment that gives bile and stools their yellowish brown color), cholesterol, and phospholipids. Bile is formed by the breakdown of hemoglobin (the protein in red blood cells that contains iron). In the gallbladder, the body concentrates the bile by absorbing some of the water it contains. Between meals, bile accumulates and is concentrated within this organ. During and after a meal, when the body begins to digest food, especially fats, the gallbladder is stimulated to contract by the release of cholestykinin in the stomach. This releases the accumulated bile, which travels through the bile duct to the small intestine. Bile is the most alkaline substance in the body.

This year, more than one million people in the United States will discover that they have gallstones. They will join an estimated 20 million Americans, approximately 10 percent of the population, who have this sometimes wretchedly painful condition. Surgical removal of the gallbladder, called cholecystectomy, is the most common surgical procedure performed in the United States. Approximately 500,000 people will undergo surgery to have their gallbladder removed this year. Gallbladder disease, in its various forms, is more likely to develop in people who are more than forty years of age and overweight.

Gallbladder disease, which may also be labeled "biliary disease," or "gallbladder attack," is most prevalent in women, although men often have this condition as well. Heredity does play a role in determining who will suffer from gallbladder problems. However, such things as diet, obesity, and age are important factors that contribute to the onset of this disease.

Large Intestine

As polite topics of conversation go, constipation, gas, diarrhea, and irritable bowel syndrome probably don't even make your list. You're probably too busy thinking about your face or figure to consider your colon. Yet you can perfect your elimination by following a few basic lifestyle rules. And if you do have a few troubles along the way, some straightforward and effective natural remedies can put you back in balance.

It's an old saying, but it's so true: "Health begins in the colon."

The large intestine is partly a storage tank for the absorption of about one liter of water daily. This tank also provides an environment for microbial fermentation. These bugs finish the job of digesting soluble fiber, starch, and undigested carbohydrates.

Anaerobic bacteria in the colon ferment the last of the food, producing short-chain fatty acids. It is largely these short-chain fatty acids that create the slightly acidic pH of fecal matter. Measurements of the amounts and proportions of the various short-chain fatty acids give an indication of the basic status of intestinal function. Elevated fecal pH (alkaline) and reduced amounts of short-chain fatty acids may indicate inadequate fiber digestion or inadequate intake of dietary fiber, which are very typical in Americans.

The Ideal Bowel Movement

The ancient lifestyle science of Ayurveda says that a healthy stool resembles a peeled, fully ripe banana in size, shape, and color. And it floats. Ayurveda says that "if your stool is sinking, you're sinking!"

Regular, bulky, soft, and comfortable bowel movements are vital to good health. But something must be seriously wrong, since 4.5 million Americans say they are constipated *most* or *all* of the time. Constipation is medically defined as passing stools less than three times a week or in low quantity.

As you might expect, like most everything else in the health field, there are major disagreements as to how you should maintain bowel function. Conventional medicine generally recommends nothing beyond increasing fluids, consuming a high-fiber diet, and getting more exercise. Complementary methods promote concepts that conventional medicine hasn't fully accepted.

A proper bowel movement depends mainly on three factors: peristalsis, fiber, and moisture.

Peristalsis is the wavelike motion that propels feces out of the large intestine. When the bowel functions properly, muscles squeeze briefly every few seconds and then relax, propelling stool toward the rectum (*transit*). So-called stimulant laxatives promote this wave. Among the best are senna leaf, cascara bark, and aloe leaf. They should be used only short term for brief episodes of acute constipation.

Fiber absorbs moisture, increasing stool size, giving the muscles in the intestinal walls something to grab on to, and making the stool softer. Natural bulk laxatives provide soluble fiber to slow intestinal motility. These include pectin from fruit, flaxseed, chia seed, and oat bran. These can be taken daily as necessary to create a soft, spongy stool. Fiber also regulates transit time by absorbing excess moisture and firming stool, slowing passage. A basic directive is to increase fiber intake (fruits, vegetables, dried legumes) to up to 35 grams per day.

Normal stool is light brown to brown. Yellow or green (an Ayurvedic sign of pitta) may indicate diarrhea (another pitta symptom) or a colon sterilized by antibiotics. Red comes from lower tract bleeding. Black stool usually means there is upper gastrointestinal tract bleeding, while tan or gray (vata signs) suggests bile duct blockage. Pancreatic insufficiency produces greasy stool. Mucus or pus, a kapha sign, indicates excess alkalinity.

The large intestine contains about 3 pounds of bacteria, including such inhabitants as *E. coli*, *Acidophilus spp.*, and other bacteria, as well as *Candida* yeast. Surprisingly, these make up about 25 to 50 percent of the dry weight of stool. In human beings, unlike cows, these bacteria don't participate much in actual digestion, although they produce the familiar stinky methane, hydrogen sulfide, and other intestinal gases as they ferment their food. As these bacteria digest our leftover food, they secrete needed nutrients, including vitamin K, vitamin B_{12}, biotin, and some amino acids.

Studies link a lack of exercise with an increased risk for colon cancer, so physicians customarily prescribe physical exercise for constipated patients. A study of lifestyle factors among 75,000 Norwegians indicated that those who walked or cycled at least four hours a week had an appreciably decreased colon cancer risk. A recent Harvard study showed that people with the highest physical activity levels had half the incidence of colon cancer of those who exercised the least.

Healthy amounts of beneficial colon bacteria (lactobacilli including *L. acidophilus,* bifidobacteria, and *E. coli*), called *probiotics,* are crucial to a healthy digestive system and good health. Lactobacilli and bifidobacteria species, in particular, have been known for a long while to be health promoters. These good bugs inhibit gut pathogens, neutralize carcinogens, maintain intestinal pH, reduce cholesterol, synthesize vitamins, and secrete enzymes that finish the breakdown of carbohydrates.

In a healthy colon, there are more than 400 species of bacteria. The probiotic microbes make up a substantial portion. In a healthy adult, bifidobacteria makes up one-quarter of the total flora. Antibiotics, chronic maldigestion, and overgrowth of invading bacteria reduce the numbers of these organisms, paving the way for infections of pathogens, including yeast. Measurement of their levels may indicate the need to supplement with "friendly bacteria" to restore these important properties.

Eating live-culture yogurt or taking high-quality probiotic supplements fortifies the colony of good bugs, preventing constipation.

Fructo-oligosaccharides (FOS) are carbohydrates that are present in some foods. We can't digest them, but that doesn't mean they're not important. Since they are not digestible, FOS pass into the colon unchanged, where they become fuel for some types of "friendly" bacteria. If you are planning to improve the health of your large intestine, it's important to make sure that the populations of these "good bugs," including acidophilus, are healthy and numerous.

According to Dr. Gaby, for some people, ingesting FOS may be an even more effective method of normalizing the intestinal flora. FOS can normalize colonic pH, so they might help to prevent colon cancer. Foods rich in FOS include burdock (3.6 percent), onion (2.8 percent), garlic (1.0 percent), rye (0.7 percent), and banana (0.3 percent).

In one study involving the administration of 8 grams of fructo-oligosaccharides per day for eight weeks to twenty-three patients with a mean age of seventy-three years, the bifidobacteria content of the feces was upped about tenfold and the pH of the stool was normalized.[4] In addition, stool consistency was improved in some cases. This benefit was also born out in another study of traveler's diarrhea. After consuming 10 grams per day of FOS, the normal healthy volunteers reported a significantly better sense of well-being during their vacation.[5]

A study from 1996 confirmed the increase in bifidobacteria with

FOS. This time, volunteers took 12.5 grams per day and controls took a placebo. The dose of FOS was well tolerated.[6]

Ruminate on These Digestive Herbs

Herbal medicine is quite effective at keeping digestion perking along, as shown in the results of one older study from Europe. Twenty-four patients received an herbal mixture containing dandelion, St. John's wort, lemon balm, calendula, and fennel. About 95 percent had total relief of colitis symptoms in fifteen days.[7]

Triphala, an Ayurvedic combination of the fruits amlaki, haritaki, and bibitaki, is the classic herbal remedy for long-term digestive benefit. It tones the intestinal walls, detoxifies the system, and promotes evacuation. It has a high tannin content, so it treats diarrhea in low doses (1 gram per day). In higher doses, it treats constipation in a very slow, gentle way, toning the walls of the gut while it works. Triphala is suitable for children and is ideal for older folks who need just a little help with regularity. For maintenance use, take 2 grams per day. As a short-term laxative, use 6 grams. An easy bowel movement will come in about eight hours. Triphala is one of the few remedies that is essentially neutral in pH, so it can be taken by just about anyone with any condition.

Turmeric root (*Curcuma longa*), an alkalizer and common curry spice, first and foremost keeps digestive inflammation (acid) under control. One of the active ingredients, curcumin, the pigment that gives turmeric its distinctive yellow color, has anti-inflammatory effects comparable to those of cortisone and phenylbutazone,[8] the standards in drugs for inflammation. Curcumin is nonsteroidal, so it has none of the ravaging side effects of steroid anti-inflammatories.[9] Curcumin also treats pain directly. Like another medicinal spice, cayenne, it depletes nerve endings of substance P, the pain receptor neurotransmitter.[10] Historically, this medicine has been used to reduce gas, a function that is now getting increasing scientific support. Curcumin stimulates gallbladder contractions, promoting better digestion.[11,12] Another compound in this herb, p-tolymethylcarbinol, increases the production of several important secretions in the digestive tract. Turmeric is widely used to improve digestion, and there is some scientific evidence that curcumin treats dyspepsia, a condition of overacidity. A double-blind placebo-controlled study with

106 patients measured the effects of 500 milligrams of curcumin taken four times daily against placebo. Seven days into the study, 87 percent of the curcumin group experienced full or partial dyspepsia symptom relief, compared to 53 percent of the placebo group.[13] With its ability to suppress inflammation, stop bleeding, and increase the stomach content of mucin, a secretion that protects against stomach acid and other digestive juices, turmeric prevents ulcerations of all types, including gastritis, peptic ulcer,[14] irritable bowel syndrome, and colitis. Take 1 to 2 grams of powdered herb in capsule form or as a spice with each meal.

Licorice root (*Glycyrrhiza uralensis*) guards digestive mucous membranes by increasing production of mucin.[15] Deglycyrrhizinated licorice root (DGL) has the glycyrrhizic acid removed. (Glycyrrhizic acid is the ingredient in licorice root associated with the possibility of occasionally increasing blood pressure and water retention.) The soothing part of the root, however, remains in DGL. One to two chewable wafers of DGL with a meal may soothe the tummy.[16] Use 1 teaspoon of chopped herb brewed as tea three times a day, or one to two chewable wafers of DGL (250 to 500 milligrams) fifteen minutes before meals and one to two hours before bedtime.

Peppermint leaf (*Mentha piperita*) is a well-known herb for tummy troubles. Enteric-coated peppermint oil works well to prevent dyspepsia. Peppermint oil is a relaxant for the muscles of the intestinal wall. Enteric coating the capsule delays the effect until the remedy is farther down in the digestive tract, as well as reducing peppermint-tasting burps. In one double-blind trial from Taiwan, four out of every five patients experienced reduced symptoms when given enteric-coated peppermint oil.[17] In 1999, a study from Germany used peppermint and caraway oils to test 223 people. The combination brought about a significant reduction in cramps.[18] A German study from February 2000 again confirmed that a combination of peppermint and caraway oils effectively reduced the speed of intestinal movement.[19] Take 1 teaspoon of chopped herb brewed as tea three times a day, or 0.2 to 0.4 milliliter of an enteric-coated capsule three times a day.

Heat Up the Digestive Fire

If you have a cold, slow stomach that is full of mucus (a kapha condition), you need to warm up your digestive tract, bring circulating blood to the digestive tissues, and increase the secretion of hot, intense (pitta) digestive juices.

Used by nearly every culture in the world, tasty, aromatic ginger root (*Zingiber officinale*) is a time-tested digestive remedy for stomach upset. Ginger's effect on motion sickness and nausea has been thoroughly proven, so it's not surprising that European practitioners use ginger in tea for indigestion. Ginger reduces spasm, absorbs and neutralizes toxins in the gastrointestinal tract, and increases the secretion of digestive juices, including bile and saliva.[20] Ginger contains ingredients that soothe the gut and aid digestion by increasing peristalsis.[21] Use 1 teaspoon of chopped herb brewed as tea three times a day.

Warming cinnamon bark (*Cinnamomum cassia*) is a mild but useful remedy for sluggish digestion. *The Complete German Commission E Monographs* (Integrative Medicine Communications, 1998), the European standard for herbal medicines, recommends cinnamon for loss of appetite, dyspeptic complaints, mild gastrointestinal spasm, bloating, and flatulence.[22] Use 1 teaspoon of chopped herb brewed as tea three times a day.

Although known exclusively as a cardiovascular medicine in Western herbalism, warming hawthorn berry is used in TCM to speed up the digestion of proteins and fats in the digestive tract.

Dr. Lark suggests a program of digestive supplements to promote the proper breakdown of food in the digestive tract.

Bromelain, derived from pineapple stem, is a proteolytic enzyme. It assists the digestive juices in breaking down proteins. If you have indigestion after consuming protein-rich foods such as red meat, poultry, milk products, and wheat, consider adding a bromelain supplement to your meal. Dr. Lark suggests 500 to 1,000 milligrams of bromelain with each meal.

Papain, another proteolytic enzyme, this time from the papaya plant, functions like bromelain. You might know it as the ingredient in commercial meat tenderizers. You can experiment to find out whether bromelain or papain works better for you. Dr. Lark favors 200 to 300 milligrams of papain with each meal. Stay away from the chewable papain tablets you see in health food stores. Your mouth is made of protein. If these were potent enough to work and you were chewing them, what would be happening to your mouth tissues?

Pancreatic enzymes are extracted from the pancreas juices of cows or pigs (although there are vegetarian versions, usually extracted from fungi, that have similar effects). They are very similar to the human enzymes produced in your pancreas. Pancreatic enzymes primarily break down carbohydrates, but they also have effects on protein and fats. The Lark program advocates 300 to 1,000 milligrams of pancreatic enzymes with each meal.

With any of these digestive enzymes, you can feel free to very gradually increase the dose to the amount that produces the most comfortable experience of complete digestion. As long as you are not experiencing any side effects (abdominal discomfort, nausea, loose stools), work up to the most effective dose.

The digestive tract is the most metabolically active place in the body. All the intense action happens there. Hot, intense fluids mix and mingle, and our food goes through its transformation. The digestive tract houses the most acid fluid in the body, and the most alkaline. The main acid reservoir and the organ that produces the most alkaline juice in a human are there. It's mighty important.

To reach the goal of Body Balance, we truly must start with the digestive tract. Everything we put in our bodies does, after all. And almost everything that has to come out comes through this very special tube. If it doesn't come out right, we have trouble. Start the process by becoming intimately aware of your digestion. Is food comfortable going in? Does food go through and come out properly? Is the timing correct? Then measure the pH of some of the parts. If required, go to a lab and have some high-tech tests of the stomach and stool done. Commit to making the changes necessary to fix what you find. To get healthy and stay healthy, it all starts here.

12

Body Balance Herbal Treatments

In a report that shocked the nation but secretly confirmed the suspicions of many mainstream physicians, David Eisenberg reported in 1993 that 54 percent of American adults had used at least one unconventional therapy in the previous year.[1] The researchers estimated that Americans made more visits to alternative healthcare practitioners in 1990, the year of the study, than to conventional primary physicians in the same period.

Then, a 1994 survey showed that over 69 percent of physicians had recommended alternative therapies to their patients at least once in the previous year.[2] A total of 23 percent of these physicians had incorporated alternatives into their own practices. And 47 percent had used alternative therapies themselves.

Four years later, John A. Astin, Ph.D., proposed that "there is no comprehensive model to account for the increasing use of alternative forms of healthcare."[3] He asked a cross-section of Americans about the use of "acupuncture, homeopathy, herbal therapies, chiropractic, massage, exercise/movement, high-dose megavitamins, spiritual healing, life-style diet, relaxation, imagery, energy healing, folk remedies, biofeedback, hypnosis, psychotherapy and art/music therapy." The study revealed that 40 percent of all subjects queried had used some form of alternative healthcare in the previous year, for a mixed bag of ailments including chronic pain, anxiety, chronic fatigue, sprains/strains, addiction, arthritis, and headaches. All socioeconomic levels had used these alternatives. Anxiety patients were twice as likely as nonanxious individuals to have used alternatives—a worthwhile thing to know, considering that herbal medicine specifically treats anxiety very effectively, without many of the disadvantages of drugs.

Significantly, only 4.4 percent of the alternative therapy users relied exclusively on alternative care. A whopping 95 percent use conventional and alternative therapies in combination.

When people don't get the results they want from conventional care, they look elsewhere. People suffering from chronic pain, anxiety, chronic fatigue, sprain/strains, addiction, arthritis, and headaches experience a high rate of failure with pharmaceutical treatment.

Reuters Health News reported in April 2000 that while alternative therapies have been gradually getting more popular over the past couple of decades, new survey findings demonstrate that nine out of ten Americans believe alternative medicine may help a wide variety of health conditions. About 74 percent of American women take dietary supplements on a daily basis, and these were by far the alternative therapy of choice. Of the respondents, 74 percent said the therapies could benefit stress relief and 67 percent said they could offset low energy. People also felt that alternative therapies could benefit joint pain and arthritis, weight gain or loss, psychological and emotional disorders, muscle building, and skin, nail, and hair conditions.

It's estimated that 75 percent of all medical sessions are for symptoms of stress-related disorders. Herbal medicine is ideally suited to these ambiguous, nonlethal problems. Patients like the results. Effective herbal medicine for these issues is relatively easy to learn about and use, although it requires a bit more time for education of and administration by the patient and has a bit of a learning curve for the physician.

While herbal medicine is branded "alternative" here in the United States, it is a time-honored profession in every other part of the world. Exhaustive systems of medicine in older cultures have extensive information regarding the clinical use of herbs, and sophisticated herbal therapeutic practices that surprise many physicians who investigate them.

Our exposure to herbal medicine in North America for the last twenty years has been but the tip of the iceberg. Physicians can learn to use herbs effectively in a clinical setting and can reap the rewards of a satisfied clientele, while seeing their rates of success improving very agreeably. Individuals can learn methods of self-care that will improve their day-to-day lives substantially.

Herbs: The Original Medicine

Humankind has been using herbal medicine since the dawn of the species to stay healthy and to treat disease. Visualize a time in the future when you haven't been concerned by even a sniffle or a tummy ache—for years. That future can become reality, and herbal medicine, properly applied and executed, can be a big part of that reality.

This is encouraging at a time when the outlook for our nation's future health is reported, by many accounts, to be bleak. In a world where health professionals admit that disease appears to be surpassing the usefulness of our medicines, fear is justifiably running high.

If you're like the average person, you long to learn what *you* can do to heal and protect yourself—not only against increasingly hardy bacteria and other infectious diseases, but also against the slow disintegration, aging, and bothersome daily symptoms that challenge the quality of so many people's lives. And you want to know that you can take the initiative to create health, strength, and vitality.

Like most of the rest of us, you're probably becoming progressively more concerned about health. You wonder about healthcare—its costs, its effectiveness. You wonder about the best ways to heal. You wonder about the way you will age and what the quality of your life will be like as the years advance. Never have Americans been more engrossed in what they can do for themselves, and never have we had so many options concerning the type of healthcare through which we can assure a good life.

This is a historic period, characterized by growing disenchantment with conventional Western medicine. The average person has become more cynical about many aspects of typical care. So, natural medicines are of overriding interest right now.

The People's Medicine

In every culture throughout the ages, herbal medicine has been self-care. Most herbal use, even today, is by people in their own homes, successfully applying folk medicine principles to treat a large variety of diseases, and to stay healthy.

Americans are ever more interested in self-care. It is becoming more and more middle-of-the-road. But self-care, in modern medicine's recent history, constitutes almost a contradiction in terms. Much of what other cultures consider "self-care" is labeled "alternative." But Americans in-creasingly are seeking alternatives.

Two studies, one done by *Consumer Reports* and the other by the University of Iowa and both reported in *The Natural Foods Merchandiser* in May 2000, show that more and more Americans are talking to their physicians about herbal remedies. When 60 percent of *Consumer Reports* readers admitted that they used herbs, a whopping 55 percent said that their doctors expressed approval. The *Consumer Reports* readers stated that they obtained better results when their herbal medicines were rec-ommended by a health professional than when they treated themselves.

James A. Duke, Ph.D., is a widely respected expert in the herbal med-icine field. He recently retired from a long career with the U.S. Department of Agriculture, during which he made numerous trips to herb-growing and -using cultures around the world, especially in South America. He is the author of *The Green Pharmacy* (Rodale, 1997), among many other authoritative herb books. According to Dr. Duke, "whole herbs are the best approach to medicine—better than what we are getting."[4] He points out that 218,000 people per year die from pharmaceuticals. "I've yet to find even 50 per year that die from herbs. Herbs are the best med-icine for whole health."

The noteworthy success of Bill Moyers's public television documen-tary *Healing and the Mind* and Dr. Andrew Weil's book *Spontaneous Healing* (Knopf, 1995) confirm our intense interest in healing alterna-tives.

Herbs have been used as medicine all over the planet for centuries, with good success in a broad range of situations. Nothing can beat mod-ern medicine for crisis care—trauma, broken bones, auto accidents, and heart attacks. But for chronic, limited, and prepathological stages of dis-ease, herbal medicine works—without a doubt. In many situations, nat-ural therapies not only work well, but are less expensive in the long run and often in the short run as well.

There are many good reasons to choose herbal medicine over con-ventional remedies in the case of most illnesses:

- Herbal medicines are often safer, while being just as effective for most common, chronic illnesses and discomforts.
- Herbal medicines are often less expensive for both the patient and the entire healthcare system (which costs us all in the long run).
- Herbal medicines often have fewer side effects, if they have any.

- Herbal medicines are more accessible.
- Herbal medicines typically deal with underlying issues, not just symptoms.

Herbal medicines help prevent health problems from developing into crises.

What Are Medicinal Herbs?

Herbs are edible plants or, from another perspective, concentrated foods. They are usually very safe, often are nutrient-rich, and are useful for their content of compounds that can nourish tissues and support the body's own healing responses. They are often quite powerful, yet are seldom habit-forming or addictive. Traditionally, herbal medicine has relied on these plants in their whole form—used in preparations that require minimal processing, including teas, powders, and food ingredients.

There is no specific definition for what constitutes a medicinal herb. We find herbs somewhere in the spectrum between food and drugs. Many herbs actually are nutritive, as food is, and essentially are used as food, consumed for their nutrient content. Other herbs have high concentrations of compounds that are not nutritive in the characteristic sense, but that nevertheless have specific actions that can influence body processes to move in the direction of healing. These herbs are used essentially for their targeted biochemical effect.

Though all herbs reside in the middle of the spectrum, some herbs lean farther toward the food side of the continuum and others are closer to the drug side. The herbs that are most foodlike, which sometimes are foods or spices, are generally the ones that are more nutritive in the characteristic sense. When parsley goes in salad, for example, it is food. But juiced and used to treat edema, it is medicine—mild medicine, but still medicine.

Closer to the drug end on the continuum is an herb such as the well-known echinacea. This medicinal herb is not nutritive like food, but contains its own unique compounds that are considered to be responsible for echinacea's supportive and stimulating effects on the immune system. Still, echinacea is far milder than a drug and requires higher doses.

On the continuum closer still to the drug end is a plant such as foxglove, from which digitalis was originally derived. This plant is very powerful, and the safety range for the dose is very narrow. A small amount of this herb could easily kill you. Traditionally, herbalists use very few herbs this close to the drug end of the spectrum, but these herbs can be valuable in the hands of a trained practitioner under the right circumstances.

So, the distinction between food and herbal medicine is a bit gray and basically arbitrary. It's a matter of dose, preparation, and convenience. Foods are composed of the same kinds of elements that make up herbs, but medicinal herbs tend to be more concentrated. If you put cinnamon in your tea for flavor, it's a food. If you use it in high doses in capsules to treat menstrual cramps, it's a medicine. The species that are chosen for use in the materia medica of the world's systems of traditional medicine tend to be those that have an appropriate balance between dose and effect. Too mild and the dose will be too high for good compliance—it's better as a food. Too concentrated, and the herb will be too dangerous to put into the hands of a patient.

We must also consider whether the plant's active ingredients will be released in the preparation that is chosen. TCM, for example, almost exclusively uses *decoctions*, a method of preparing herbs as soups or strong, concentrated teas. Therefore, they tend to favor herbs that have water-soluble active ingredients—herbs that centuries of experience has shown will be effective medicine when prepared in this way.

Herbs Versus Drugs

Pharmacology has its roots, so to speak, in herbalism. Many drugs, still today, are extracted from plants or are synthesized versions of phytochemicals. There are several important reasons why herbs may be a healthier and more sensible choice for treating a great many health conditions and for enhancing existing health. So what's the difference between drugs and herbal preparations?

Our Bodies Know Herbs

The first great benefit of herbs is that our bodies know what to do with them and with the component chemicals they contain. Medicinal herbs contain essentially the same phytochemicals as foods. Our bodies recognize them because we have been consuming compounds like these for millennia. All around the globe, in every culture, humans evolved being exposed to plant foods and the building blocks of plants. Our bodies know how to assimilate, digest, and excrete waste from plant compounds. Our bodies do not react negatively to most plant compounds. They aren't foreign.

On the other hand, drugs are new to the human body. They've been around for only a couple of generations, and some drugs now being prescribed have been on the market for only a year. These compounds are largely unfamiliar to our systems, and our bodies don't know as well what to do with these unrecognizable foreigners because they haven't had millennia to evolve specific adaptations for dealing with these substances. Drugs are more likely to create side effects for this and other reasons.

In *Spontaneous Healing,* Dr. Andrew Weil claims drug toxicity is "the most common sin of commission of conventional medicine today" and says, "In whatever form and for whatever reason you take drugs, you are increasing the workload on your liver, since it is the task of the liver to metabolize most foreign substances." Therefore, most herbs are appropriate for long-term use, while most drugs are not.

Herbs Still Have All Their Parts

The second great benefit of herbs, when used traditionally in their whole form, is the action of a large collection of complementary components. All plant medicines can be shown to have from dozens to thousands of component ingredients, which act synergistically to enhance health. Some of these components are considered primary active ingredients, others complement and support the actions of those active ingredients, some are nutritive, still others are antidotes to still others, and so on. The whole plant complex retains compounds that may mitigate any deleterious effects of active ingredients. All of these phytochemicals act in different ways or through slightly different metabolic pathways, in concert with each other, to create the desired effect. For this reason, most traditional herbalists consider the strength of herbal medicine to be in the use of these whole herbs. As medicines, whole herbs are both more effective and safer for the roster of all their complementary constituents.

Conversely, while drugs are valuable for relieving symptoms and are sometimes necessary, the broader action of herbs may be superior for restoring underlying health. The conventional approach of isolating an active ingredient from a plant (for example, the salicylates that became aspirin were first isolated from meadowsweet) creates striking and highly focused activity that is much more likely to produce side effects. Herbs typically contain multiple chemical variants of any given active compound. These subtly different molecules often act over an extended range of time, absorption pathways, and elimination mechanisms. Since one exclusive metabolic pathway is not overburdened by large amounts of a single, often foreign molecule and the action of the metabolites is spread out over several pathways, the cumulative effect is likely to be highly effective, albeit possibly slower in action, and far less likely to cause negative reactions, as the different components complement each other. For this same reason, herbs are less likely to produce tolerance. Drugs may prove to be less effective for long-term conditions that require gentle sustained action.

Medicinal herbs selected by traditional peoples tend to be balanced by nature, and when an herb is used in its whole form, side effects are almost never an issue. Many traditional herbalists believe that there is an innate ecological wisdom in the way a given plant is composed, having evolved to contain that unique and specific combination of components.

Although herbs contain chemical compounds that have biological actions, they are more than "drug delivery systems." The interplay of this rainbow of related components and associated factors creates a much different dynamic than the large doses of a single molecule. The flip side of this is that natural products are, by nature, unpredictable. It is impossible to know the exact percentage of each potential active component in any given dose of herb. It is simply too complex. Coupled with the natural variation in plant samples, this creates a concern that it would be difficult to assess the proper dose or to achieve consistent results in any given case. While this is a valid point, this turns out to be a minimal issue in practical reality. Ethnic herbalists have commercial supplies of herbs that were procured and processed by professionals. These herbs were evaluated "organoleptically"—that is, by the senses—for consistency and potency. In point of fact, herbalists find little significant variation in clinical potency in herbs from established sources.

In addition, an herb is made up of a lower percentage of active ingredient than is a drug. Herbs are inherently more dilute, thanks to the presence of other plant material, such as fiber, as well as other phytochemical constituents. This promotes safety and ease of use in self-care. Of course, the trade-off can be compliance when the dose of the dilute herb becomes cumbersome.

Herbs Reestablish Health to the Whole

Herbs have, throughout history, been used in the context of an organized system of natural medicine, which aims to correct the causal pathology, usually involving healing actions on the interconnected systems and organs of the whole body with the ultimate goal being to restore health and equilibrium. While herbs can treat symptoms quite effectively, this is not the focal point of the traditional systems of healthcare.

This difference in orientation does not just arise out of the biological differences between herb chemistry and drug chemistry, but from *the paradigm in which they are used*. When we discuss this topic, we must separate herbs, which can be used in a druglike way (hence the designation "green drugs"), from the concepts of holism, which underpin all traditional systems of medicine in which herbalism plays a part.

Typically herbalists, especially those trained in a system from an established tradition such as Ayurveda or TCM, are not concerned merely with dulling symptoms, which may be an element of therapy initially for the patient's immediate relief, but with restoring proper function and homeostasis. In herbalism, it is preferable to eliminate a symptom by eliminating its cause rather than by merely masking the symptom. It is also desirable to gently activate the body's own performance rather than to replace the missing function. For example, in herbal medicine it is preferable to nourish and direct the body to return to normal hormonal production and regulation, rather than to simply replace hormones that are missing or insufficient.

Herbs can be used as "treatment," but they are used more effectively to boost and maintain health. Herbs excel in this area, and herbalism is at its best when used for this purpose. Many herbs are useful even when you are well. In traditional cultures, people take the majority of the herbs they consume when they are well, in an effort to avoid disease.

Herbs are less convenient than drugs. When you have a headache, you can take two ibuprofen tablets and have your headache go away fast. Brewing two cups of willow bark tea takes longer. The herb takes a while to steep. It takes longer to work. It doesn't taste very good. On average, herbs do take longer to work than drugs, and they require more effort and responsibility. However, herbs are effective, cost-efficient, nontoxic, and noninvasive. The personal effort required to use them is worth it.

Chinese Herbal Combinations

TCM is probably the most intricate system of herbal medicine in the world. Formulas with a dozen or more ingredients are not uncommon. The science of combining herbs is deep and complex in TCM.

The gradual maturity of formulation followed the accumulation, over the centuries, of an escalating number of herbs in the materia medica and a steady deepening in the perceptions of the process of disease.

Herbs are combined to increase therapeutic benefit, reduce side effects, encompass complex clinical presentations, and modify the actions of the therapeutic herbs themselves. Currently, most TCM formulas contain six to twelve ingredients.

Is Every Herb Safe?

Yes, most herbs are safe. But not all are. There *is* potential to do damage with herbs; there is no doubt about that. You've probably heard the adage "the dose makes the poison." There are a handful of herbs, used, in traditional cultures, only by trained herbalists, that are naturally so potent that they could be injurious if misused.

Nevertheless, it is clear that most herbs, because they are so dilute and because the active components are spread over such a broad range of action, are safe. Many herbs, like foods, can be taken in as high a quantity as you care to reasonably eat because no matter how much you take of them, they will only nourish you. Adverse herb events are much rarer than adverse drug events, even though negative herb scenarios are getting far more attention in the media these days.

The consensus of clinical experience of most herbalists, naturopathic physicians, and other natural health practitioners supports that. Time after time, these practitioners report that just 1 to 2 percent of all their patients experience mild reactions.

In *The Medicine Garden*, a public broadcasting radio documentary produced by David Freudberg, Robert Temple, who evaluates drugs for the Food and Drug Administration (FDA), says that's hard to believe. In typical clinical studies of drugs, he says, it's common to see 25 to 30 percent of users having adverse reactions. "It's inconceivable that plant-derived materials are not associated with the same kinds of side effects," he charges. But Andrew Weil has counted on herbal remedies for the last twenty years in his practice and calculates that for every prescription drug he suggests, he recommends forty to fifty plant products. This has never produced a single serious negative reaction, he says, just, at worst, a couple of rashes and a couple of upset stomachs. The patient is told to discontinue use. That rate, he says, is utterly insignificant compared to that for drugs. The risks of toxicity from drugs are significant, both in number and kinds of reactions, "which include death and permanent disability," he says in *The Medicine Garden*.

Pharmacognosy

When traditional healers study and teach about herbs, it is always in the larger context of the entire traditional healing system in which that style of herbal medicine matured. Herbs are used, in those systems, against the background of a person's entire life and are supplemented by other elements of the lifestyle. Many American herbalists studied herbal medicine within one of these perspectives, such as Native American herbalism, and are considered traditional herbalists.

There is a different way that herbs are studied academically, included in the paradigm of conventional scientific medicine, called "pharmacognosy." Pharmacognosy applies the scientific principles of modern knowledge to herbal medicine; much the way pharmacology is studied. Essentially, plant medicines are analyzed for their components, which are studied for their individual effects. This is accomplished outside of the context that gives herbal medicine its life and meaning, its richness of texture.

While pharmacognosy is valuable and gives insight about the actions of herbs, forming another lens through which to view the plants, it is not herbalism. Utilizing pharmacognosy requires that the herbs be plucked out of the healing system in which they arose, leaving behind all of the accompanying wisdom, scrutiny, intuition, and judiciousness of the system that makes it so useful, understandable, and safe in its culture of origin.

Orthodox scientists like this approach to herbs. Herbs, then, are treated like drugs. But since traditional herbs are not drugs, they often don't fit in very well, and they suffer in the interpretation.

Medical professionals sometimes complain that they cannot understand herbs or see any benefit to them. This may be because herbal medicine is complicated, has a huge materia medica, often uses extensive polyherb formulas, and varies from culture to culture. For example, determining that an herb can kill a pathogen in a test tube may shed no light on how the herb performs clinically. The herb may instead effect global changes in the host that make the host reject the pathogen, for example.

It's important to understand that *pharmacognosy does not equal herbal medicine*—at least not the scope of traditional herbal medicine. Pharmacognosy is basically the pharmacological analysis of herbs—valuable, but not complete. Pharmacognosists frequently view herbs merely as diluted drugs. While that may be true from a certain limited point of view, herbalism can be appreciated from a number of levels. Furthermore, pharmacognosists may insist that medicinal herbs cannot be considered foods or nutritional supplements, for anything used to treat disease or affect health must conform to the definition of the word "drug." Pharmacognosists also usually see no difference between natural and synthetic substances, although this view has been called into question recently with some noteworthy examples, such as the minor chemical distinction between natural and synthetic beta-carotene and its significance in cancer treatment.

This view trickles down from science to the consumer. When herbs are plucked out of their traditional milieu and separated from all of the traditional methodologies that surrounded them, they become merely abstract substances to be applied like any drug.

This tendency to expect herbs to act like drugs has caused big misinterpretations in our culture lately. As herbal medicine boomed in the 1990s, marketers convinced the public that herbs were nontoxic remedies that could be expected to act like drugs—for example, they would cure depression, lower cholesterol, or blunt arthritis pain. Of course, stripped from the traditional healing systems, they could not live up to the hype. Mass disappointment ensued.

Understanding acid-alkaline balance is a window into applying traditional herbal medicine in a consistent, holistic way.

Modern "Global Herbalism"

It is generally believed that the flowering of modern medicine began with Descartes, during the European Renaissance. This is probably true from the philosophical perspective, as this was the first time that a mass movement of people began to think of the human mind as separate from the human body. It was the beginning of the end for "holism," the core idea of human identity theretofore.

Really, what we think of as conventional medicine had its beginnings as recently as the 1940s, when some remarkable changes took place in mainstream medicine, among them the introduction of antibiotics and major tranquilizers. Radical advances in pharmacology and surgery have dominated medicine in our culture to this day.

Most of the states in the United States had both natural and conventional medical boards into the 1940s. But natural methods, already on the decline, just could not compete with the astonishing technological progress in antibiotics, tranquilizers, and surgical techniques. Conventional medical practitioners, called "allopaths" by some, operating under a rationalist, or mechanistic, paradigm, have dominated American medicine, and the whole of Western medicine, since that time.

Despite this, herbal medicine, and a wide variety of other modalities, did not quite die out in America. During the last quarter of the twentieth century, things began to slowly heat up.

In 1978, we saw the founding of the American Holistic Medical Association. The thrust of this organization was that all standard conventional techniques would still be applied in practice; that there would be a greater emphasis upon behavioral medicine and acupuncture, and possibly homeopathy; and that there would also be an emphasis on the spiritual dimension of health.

Even by 1991, the term "alternative medicine" was not yet widely used. *Time* magazine reported on the growing trend in its November 4, 1991, issue. The article stated: "It reflects a growing dissatisfaction with conventional medicine."

Congress established a national Office of Alternative Medicine early in the 1990s.

The 1993 Eisenberg study indicated that 34 percent of Americans reported "using at least one unconventional therapy in the past year." Conspicuously, American citizens were spending more out of their pocket on alternative therapies than they spent out of their pocket for all hospitalization and primary care. They were not telling their medical doctors.

Historically, herbalists studied regional systems of herbalism, bonding intricately with the prevailing worldview of the native culture. That, in and of itself, was a lifetime of study. A Chinese herbalist, say, whether studying in China or in America, had no need to go further than the historical and contemporary teachings of TCM to have an incredibly full plate. Typically an apprentice would study with a master herbalist locally and would become an expert in the plants and style of medicine in that locale.

In these stable ancient cultures, an apprentice was taught by a master and then became a master and had his own apprentice, and so it went generation after generation. They experimented, they made their own contributions to the field, they passed on the knowledge, and the knowledge continued to expand. But the systems didn't mix very much.

In fact, any place that people live on the surface of the earth puts you within a day's walk of enough herbs to treat all the ills that you might ever come across in the civilization of that particular area. Most native ethnic herbalists have repertoires of about 2,000 different substances—meaning they not only can prescribe them appropriately, but can identify them in the wild, harvest them, process them properly, and prepare them for the best effect.

Over this quarter century, herbal medicine was advancing in every country and was beginning to rub shoulders with established medicine. As herbalists, previously isolated in ethnic systems, began to study each other's methods and to read each other's literature, they became anxious to try anything that would expand their repertoire and help their patients.

Global herbalism was born.

Today, the ethnic divisions are rapidly fading. Herbalists are sharing each other's paradigms and materia medica. This has provided a strong, diverse base of knowledge.

Thanks to global herbalism, the best things from around the entire world are available to everyone now, allowing us to practice a style of herbal medicine that offers incredible diversity. The evolution of this kind of herbal medicine requires that the herbalist learn about botanical medicines from all over the globe, not just about those indigenous to the area.

In the last five to ten years, we have been able to do things with natural healing, and especially with herbal medicine, that we could only dream of before that. It's become a very small world. We can get herbs from anywhere, things we could only hope to read about in a book ten years ago—the best of everything from China, India, Africa—things that are remarkably effective, even high powered, and that rival much of what conventional medicine has to offer. Modern methods of communication and transportation have made available any herb we might know about, from anywhere on the planet, at a moment's notice. We can call China on the phone and have an herb air-freighted to us the next day. Today we can create previously unheard of combinations that may be much more effective medicine than a single herb or a combination limited to one ethnic system.

These benefits of the globalization of herbal medicine compensate for what has been lost by the fragmenting of traditional ethnic communities—the downside of increased transportation and communication.

In many places today, that stable and ancient system has broken down. In some areas, there are no masters to study with anymore. North America is unfortunately one of those areas. Much of the herbal medicine originally developed here died with the native peoples. There certainly are some experts who continue to study what was recorded, and to some extent that knowledge has been saved. But there aren't many people left who know the indigenous native plants of this area. So much of what North American herbalists know is a fusion of what herbalists from other older, foreign systems have learned in the context of their own healing systems. Fortunately, because each of the systems has so much to offer, this blending has yielded a powerful brand of medicine that is even greater than the individual systems.

TCM doctors Harriet Beinfield and Efrem Korngold observe in *Between Heaven and Earth: A Guide to Chinese Medicine* that while the doctor in Western medicine is essentially a mechanic, in Eastern healing philosophies such as Chinese medicine, the doctor is like a gardener. A gardener is not a "fixer" of things so much as an ally; he nurtures, promotes, enhances, and works with the garden, *but does not try to control it*. A garden is a system that's alive, and the rule of Chinese medicine is to cultivate life. By contrast, one of the rules of the Cartesian doctrine came to be to prevent death at all costs. In the East, healers seek to make the body well; in the West, we seek to keep it alive. There is a difference.

Gardeners and mechanics use different implements. When concepts of health, disease, the body, and medicine became fixed in this manner, the contents of the medicine chest transformed. Natural therapies obviously are not based on the Cartesian model. Quite the opposite; they are based on holistic principles, meaning the whole is considered in the assessment of health or illness and the treatment of disease, and reinforcement of the host internally is as or more important than eradication of disease-causing agents externally.

Body Balance Herbs

Just like we did with food, we can begin to get a general sense of which medicinal herbs will move the pH in specific directions. Some herbs will acidify some people, while others will alkalinize. Herbs, even more than foods, are chemically complex. So, in the long run, you need to select an herbal program and follow it for a while to test it out. Here are some herbs that I, as well as many herbalists, including Dr. Kartar of the New Cleanse, believe will push pH in the direction you need it to go:

- Acidifying herbs—Cayenne and other chilies, hawthorn berry, pond lily bulb, strawberry leaf
- Alkalinizing herbs—Alfalfa, amla fruit, bhumy amalaki, black pepper, cinchona bark, gotu kola, licorice, nettle, pau d'arco bark, thyme leaf, turmeric, yucca root

Remember, most Americans are too acid, so you will probably have the best results with the herbs in the alkalinizing column.

Herbs are becoming popular again. Americans, in record numbers, are turning to this basic form of healthcare. But people are confused. We have been without a coherent system of natural health management for almost a century. We have a lot of herbs, but very little herbalism. Gradually, this situation is changing, but it will be a while before we reach the level of familiarity of a system such as Ayurveda. Modern global herbalism is becoming the way of the future. As we gain access to the accumulated wisdom of centuries of folk and academic experimentation and come to an understanding of the insights of our forefathers, we are becoming able to apply these precepts in the modern world.

Herbal medicine has been the medicine of humankind since the dawn of humanity. Every culture has worked out a systemic way to use herbs so they have maximum effect for each individual. The explanations have varied, but they had in common the idea of differential diagnosis, a methodical approach to individualizing treatment to each person and each condition. The older systems did not have chemical knowledge adequate to utilize pH concepts. But now that knowledge is at hand.

Using herbs will get you healthy and keep you healthy. Using herbs along with the modern understanding of pH will be even more effective. This graceful weaving of old and new has created an even more successful approach to enjoying a healthy and happy life.

13

Body Balance Home Remedies

Food has been the medicine of humanity since the dawn of time. Many herbs that we associate only with seasoning food are, in fact, potent herbal medicines.

The distinction between herbal food and herbal medicine is actually quite subjective. There is a wide area of overlap with the two categories. If you think of all the plants we consume, for whatever purpose, as being on a spectrum, from food on one end to medicine on the other, you will see what I mean. On the food end would be plants such as potatoes and carrots—potentially medicinal, but mild and safe. The other end of the spectrum would contain medicine plants such as opium poppy and foxglove, the source of digitalis—definitely not food, but clearly serious medicine.

The gray area is in the middle. Take echinacea. None of us would consider sitting down to a delicious bowl of echinacea soup. Yuck. But you could. And it would be safe. How about parsley? In a salad, it's a food. Used as a juice to treat edema, it's a medicine.

The truth is, herbal medicines have about the same chemical components as food plants. Herbal medicines are just selected from plants that have greater concentrations of active ingredients, making them more convenient to use.

European herbal medicine, the tradition from which contemporary American herbalism mainly derives, does not see much overlap between food plants and herbal medicines. Foods you eat, spices you add to food to make it taste better, and herbal medicine you take in a tincture. Asian medical systems, however, make no distinction between the two. Food is just less concentrated herbal medicine, and every meal is viewed as a chance to get in more healing herbs. In fact, the Chinese word for the medicinal brew that people use daily to maintain their health means "soup."

The complex cuisines of China and India began thousands of years ago as recipes to get healing herbs and foods into people. Gradually, as the process evolved, complicated mixtures of food ingredients, herbal medicines, and flavorings coalesced into a tasty amalgam that warms the soul, heals the body, and pleases the palate.

For example, Indian food typically starts with a combination, a *masala*, of onions, garlic, ginger, and various other spices, selected for their medicinal virtues and taste. Since many of these herbs can cause gas, additional herbs, such as fennel or coriander seed, are added to counteract that tendency. Ginger and mustard, for example, speed up the digestive process, allowing the meal to be efficiently processed and moved through the digestive tract.

Although the list of herbal medicine foods is huge, following is a selection of remedies that are easy to find and particularly effective.

Parsley to the Rescue

The carrot and parsley family (*Umbelliferae*), in particular, is a huge source of edible plants and good-tasting medicines. These plants grow all over the world and are used in a broad range of cultures. This group of plant medicines has unusual chemistry, so they have made their way into the kitchens and medicine chests of many native medical systems. The seeds are typically the medicinal part, but various parts are used, depending on the plant. Some well-known members of this family include parsley, coriander (cilantro is coriander greens), fennel, anise, cumin, and dill.

Plants in this family contain compounds that act like calcium channel blockers, benefiting angina. They generally have estrogenic action, especially the seeds. The popular Chinese herb dong quai is in this family. In addition, these parsley relatives are prized around the world for treating intestinal gas, a property herbalists call "carminative."

Dill

For gas, dill seed is for children what fennel seed is for adults. Called "the secret of British nannies," dill is the active ingredient in the famous "gripe water," the colic remedy used around the world in the British Empire.

Dill seed is truly miraculous for infant colic. It can save a parent's sanity. For infant colic, brew 2 tablespoons of dill seed in 1 cup of water, cool, sweeten, put in a bottle or dropper, and serve to the screaming baby. You will carry a sleeping tyke back to bed. For adults, dill, along with fennel, treats heartburn.

Dill promotes menstruation, so it can be used to encourage the start of a late period.

For milder effects, use dill weed instead of dill seed. In a pinch, fennel and dill can be interchanged.

Fennel

In my personal clinical experience, I would pick fennel seed as the premier carminative in the world, especially for adults. Literally, I have never seen a case of painful gas that was not relieved by fennel seeds, provided, of course, that the dose was high enough.

Fennel contains creosol and alpha-pinene, substances that loosen lung mucus and help clear the chest, benefiting asthma.[1] Recent research shows that this spice also lowers blood pressure.[2]

Fennel has been used for centuries to promote lactation, which makes sense from what we now know about its hormonal action. It will also hasten the onset of menstruation. As a bonus, it increases libido.

For gas, try chewing 1 tablespoon of the tasty seeds, or brew a tea made with 1 tablespoon of seeds per cup of water. You can use the powdered seeds as a seasoning or in capsules.

Of course, you can also steam the stalk as a delicious celery-like vegetable. The properties of the stalk are similar to but milder than those of the seed.

Parsley

Ever notice that green sprig of garnish at the edge of your plate? Usually discarded, that parsley is one powerful herbal medicine.

While the seeds, leaf, and root of this plant are all used as food, the main herbal uses come from the leaf.

Parsley, as you might expect, is a source of phytoestrogens, so it has potential for treating osteoporosis and amenorrhea, and for promoting lactation. It has a long history of use with the urinary system, particularly in treating bladder infections. Research shows that it is a diuretic.[3] Parsley treats angina. Crushed and applied to a bruise, it heals. It inhibits the release of histamine, so is useful for allergies and hives. It prevents and treats kidney stones.[4]

Parsley is a treasure trove of vitamins and minerals. It is a rich source of boron and fluorine, critical minerals for bone health. It contains three and a half times as much vitamin C as oranges and twice as much calcium as broccoli. Three ounces of parsley contain about 3 milligrams of boron, the dose suggested for bone health. In my clinical experience, a dose of about 2 ounces per day of parsley juice treats edema very well. Because parsley is a rich source of alkalinizing calcium, magnesium, and potassium, it is an effective treatment for cramps, such as leg cramps.[5]

Parsley leaf is widely available in capsule form, both as a single herb and in combination. It works well as a digestive aid combined with turmeric. A typical dose is 2 to 9 grams per day, but of course, this herb is very safe at any dose.

More Herbal Medicine Foods

Your kitchen brims with medicinal foods. The simplest spices can be powerful weapons against disease. Some of these tasty spices can find their way right onto your dinner plate and into your health program. One of the best ways to get large quantities of alkalinizing foods into your diet is to use these concentrated nutrient sources in the delicious dishes you and your family eat every day.

Basil Leaf

Originally from India, basil has grown to great popularity around the world. There are many varieties of this spicy leaf, but they all basically have the same medicinal qualities. One famous variety, "holy" basil, is a standout in the Ayurvedic pharmacopoeia.

Historically, basil has been used as a digestive aid, to relieve gas and speed digestion, and to warm up and mobilize stiff arthritic joints. It is a pungent herb that increases body heat. It is used to treat respiratory conditions such as the flu, and to lower fever by sweating. Since it's also an expectorant, it can be used for conditions such as emphysema and asthma.

A member of the mint family, basil contains antibacterial compounds.[6] Recent studies have shown that basil appears to prevent cancer.[7]

Basil lowers blood pressure. It contains antiviral compounds. A common folk remedy for warts is to apply crushed basil directly to the wart.

Use basil liberally in food, such as pesto, or brew it into a tea. For a headache, try chewing several fresh basil leaves.

Black Pepper

Black pepper is known only as a humble condiment in the United States, but in Asia, it is considered to be the foremost detoxifier and antiaging herb.

Black pepper is a warming digestive remedy that has a carminative action. It increases circulation and lowers blood pressure. It also contains compounds that prevent osteoporosis.

While black pepper has been esteemed as a detoxifier, particularly in Ayurveda, recent research has begun to bear this out. At least in rats, pepper seems to increase the release of carcinogens through the liver, reducing cancer.[8] Piperine, a main active ingredient, protects against liver damage almost as well as milk thistle.[9] This alkaloid is also getting a reputation for increasing bioavailability and absorption of nutrients.[10] For example, in one recent study, scientists measured the absorption of turmeric's active ingredients. Administering the turmeric along with piperine increased bioavailability by 154 percent and reduced the absorption time by half.[11]

Black pepper reduces free radicals. It is an antioxidant and prevents the depletion of glutathione. It also prevents the destruction of other antioxidants, such as vitamin A.[12] Pepper is used in Ayurveda to release sinus congestion.[13]

Black pepper is available in health food stores as a supplement. Use 50 milligrams per day or more of an extract standardized to piperine.

Use black pepper as a culinary spice. An excellent Ayurvedic preparation for sinus congestion is to boil ten peppercorns in milk, strain, and drink.

Fenugreek Seed

Fenugreek seed is getting a lot of attention lately for its many medicinal virtues. This little legume is a very rich source of soluble fiber.

Fenugreek seed is a very effective diabetes treatment, promoting substantial reductions in blood sugar, both from its fiber content and the presence of other metabolically active components. Fenugreek seed lowers total cholesterol, while increasing high-density lipoprotein (HDL), the healthy lipoprotein. It contains very high amounts of choline and beta-carotene, both of which have been linked to Alzheimer's prevention and treatment. In addition, it contains the phytoestrogen diosgenin, which has gotten attention lately for its role in preventing breast cancer.

Use fenugreek liberally as a spice in foods. The dose shown in experiments to control blood sugar is high, about 100 grams per day. That's a lot of fenugreek, which can be bitter in those quantities. In scientific studies, the fenugreek seed was often baked into flat bread or cooked into a soup. I have had good success with soaking the seeds overnight to soften them and then just chowing them down, perhaps mixed with a mild food like oatmeal.

However, one recent study showed significant reduction in total cholesterol and triglycerides with a dose of 2.5 grams twice daily, a dose that can easily be taken in capsules.[14] Fenugreek can be found in the health food store as whole powdered herb in capsules or as a standardized extract.

With such a rich selection of healing foods to choose from, there should be little problem putting together a menu of delicious medicinal recipes. Use these foods daily. You'll like making your cupboard into your medicine chest.

Nettle

That's right, the stinging nettles you dig out as a pesky weed are a good healing food. They are quite edible and tasty. The sting is neutralized when the plant is dried or cooked. When prepared like spinach, nettles have a similar, but saltier, taste. Please don't harvest this vegetable unless you know what you are doing, since the sting, before being neutralized, is painful.

Nettle is a favorite of European herbalists, who use it as a general nutritive tonic, similar to the way alfalfa is used in American herbalism. In addition, it has been historically used to treat childhood eczema and respiratory conditions, and to strengthen the circulatory tissue.[15] Recently, nettle has been getting attention in natural healing circles for the treatment of allergic rhinitis (hay fever).[16]

You can find nettle in health food stores in capsule form. Most people find that about 2 grams will relieve an allergy attack.

Thyme

Thyme contains antiaging chemicals. Historically, this herb has been used for headaches.

Thyme is known as a general antimicrobial, especially for bacterial infection, and as an expectorant that also treats fever, so it is a well-known treatment for diseases such as the flu. One ingredient, thymol, has antiviral properties and is also antispasmodic, so it is used to treat headaches and cramps.[17]

Use thyme as a tea or gargle.

Foods for Healing Specific Conditions

Body-balancing foods can be quite effective in treating specific diseases. Ayurveda, in particular, uses food as a safe medicine to benefit particular conditions. Since food is a much less concentrated source of healing phytochemicals than herbs, and much more dilute than drugs, you must use it in a much more concentrated way to get noticeable results in a reasonable time frame. Don't be surprised that the doses of some of these therapeutic foods seem a little high—they are the amounts required to get the job done.

Since many, if not most, disease conditions in modern life stem from excess acidity, you will find that many of these healing foods are detoxifying, a nod toward getting the acid wastes out of the body efficiently, as well as cooling and anti-inflammatory, a step toward suppressing the inflammation caused by the buildup of excess acid in the tissues.

Acne

Green vegetables are an important tool in the treatment of inflamed skin. Considered the most "cooling," or anti-inflammatory, of foods, they are even more cooling when used raw. Any green vegetables—spinach, celery, cucumber, even green beans—will work.

It may be the high magnesium content in the chlorophyll (the green pigment), which is known to cool inflammation, or some yet-to-be-identified component, possibly bioflavonoids, but high amounts of green vegetables will bring acute acne, psoriasis, and dermatitis under control quickly, say natural healing experts. Because it is easy to fill up quickly on fibrous raw green vegetables, juicing is a good choice for getting in large amounts of the active ingredients. Try a couple of tall glasses of cucumber or celery juice per day.

Backache

Turmeric curbs inflammation. One of the active ingredients, curcumin, the pigment that gives turmeric its distinctive yellow color, has anti-inflammatory effects comparable to cortisone and phenylbutazone, the standard in drugs for inflammation. Curcumin is nonsteroidal, so it has none of the ravaging side effects of steroid anti-inflammatories.

Curcumin also treats pain directly. Like another medicinal spice, cayenne, it depletes nerve endings of substance P, the pain receptor neurotransmitter.

Turmeric has historically been used as an external poultice for sprains and sore joints.

Willow bark is widely used in Europe for the treatment of low back pain. An Israeli study from 2000 confirmed this benefit. The 191 back pain sufferers took an extract containing either 120 or 240 milligrams of salicin per day. The extract was considerably more effective than the placebo in this blinded trial. The higher dose was quite a bit more effective. The responses in the high-dose group were evident after only one week of treatment.[18]

Bad Breath

Ever eat in an Indian restaurant? Did you notice the dish of fennel seeds by the exit? You just ate a meal of beans, onion, and garlic, which produce intestinal gas. Grab those fennel seeds, pop them in your mouth, and chew them slowly. They will lessen the gas and sweeten the breath.

Cold and Flu

Four tea herbs really stand out in the fight against cold and flu. Astragalus root (*Astragalus membranaceus* or *huang qi*) is renowned for its ability to enhance the immune system. Although it is preferred for long-term prevention, astragalus can be used for acute cold and flu. Since this herb is a building tonic, it is used primarily in chronic colds, character-ized by a weak voice, a serious aversion to cold with an inability to warm up, a pale face, and body aches, but will produce improvement in just about any case. People with chronic colds are usually alkaline. According to TCM, astragalus strengthens the lungs. Families in China often add astragalus to the family teapot during the cold season so that everyone can get a daily immune boost.

Astragalus abounds in the scientific literature. Many studies have proven its ability to enhance immune function, including activity against Coxsackie virus, a flulike virus that mainly affects children. This herb contains im-mune-enhancing polysaccharides similar to those found in echinacea and shiitake mushroom.

Unlike most Chinese herbs, astragalus actually tastes pretty good as a tea, with a velvety texture and a buttery taste.

Isatidis root (*Isatis tinctora* or *ban lan gen*) is considered to be synergis-tic with astragalus, and the two are commonly used in combination. Where astragalus is warming, isatidis is a cooling herb, so it is used to re-duce fever. Combination products are widely available. Isatidis is a broad-spectrum antimicrobial, with activity against many types of viruses and bacteria. According to TCM, it also strengthens the lungs. It does not taste great, but in a cold crisis, you should be able to stomach it mixed with astragalus.

The pleasant-tasting and sweet-smelling honeysuckle flower (*Lonicera japonica* or *jin yin hua*), when dried and brewed into a tea, is used in TCM to treat acute fever and sore throat. This cooling herb also strengthens the lungs, and it actually tastes good.

Chrysanthemum flower (*Chrysanthemum morifolium* or *ju hua*) is the flower you see at the florist, but get it from your herbalist, please. This cooling herb treats fever and red, dry, swollen eyes. It strengthens the lungs. This herb also has immune-enhancing properties. Chrysanthemum kills many pathogenic bacteria, including strep. In TCM, chrysanthemum is often combined with honeysuckle for a delicious, effective drink, especially for inflammation (acid pH).

Cough

Marshmallow root (*Althaea officinalis*) excels in cough treatment. The modern campfire food is a descendent of an old-fashioned medicinal candy made from marshmallow herb. But marshmallow has been used medicinally since the time of ancient Greece, and Roman physicians suggested marshmallow for irritated tissues.

Marshmallow root contains very high levels of mucilage, made of large sugar molecules, which have a soothing effect on mucous membranes. Modern herbalists therefore recommend marshmallow primarily for relieving respiratory problems, such as coughs. Marshmallow quells irritation and associated dry cough, according to European authorities.[19]

While scientific evidence is sparse, marshmallow did look good in one experiment in cats. In a German journal article, scientists reported that the concentrated plant sugars (polysaccharides) from the root were about as effective as a standard drug in stopping the cough reflex.[20] Marshmallow is thought to be entirely safe. It is approved for food use.

Mullein (*Verbascum thapsus*) is a common wildflower that grows almost anywhere. You have likely seen it growing along the roadside. Mullein is listed in the herbal literature as an expectorant and demulcent (soothing) herb. Both the leaf and flower are used. Contemporary herbalists recommend hot mullein tea for coughs, sore throats, and other respiratory irritations, and it is approved in Europe for that use.

Mullein rarely produces striking effects, but it can soothe a sore throat and bring some temporary relief. Like marshmallow, mullein has high mucilage content. Its actions may also be from the mucus-loosening saponins it contains. Herbalists often say that mullein is most effective when combined with herbs with similar qualities, such as yerba santa leaf and elecampane root. Mullein seems to be antiviral. Interestingly, recent research indicates the possibility that mullein may be active against herpes and the flu.[21,22] Mullein leaves and flowers are on the American Generally Recognized as Safe (GRAS) list.

Earache

I've raised three children. None of them has ever had an ear infection. Earaches may resolve themselves, but they sure can make our children miserable. None of us would like our child to suffer so. Fortunately, there is no need for all that misery. Herbal ear oils (herbs infused into a vegetable oil base) are the pillar of a natural treatment program for acute earache. First on the list is garlic. The classic herbal ear treatment, it is rapidly effective. Fill the ear with the liquid, insert a cotton ball and tape in place, and send the child to bed. In the morning, the aged garlic will have penetrated, and the earache will be gone.

Another effective home remedy is the Chinese herb *ma huang* (*Ephedra sinensis*) used externally in the ear. Brew it up as a very strong tea, let it cool, and apply a few drops in the ear. It will open the ear canal. Follow with a few drop of glycerine, which will pull the fluid out of the ear once the canal is open.

An Israeli study done in 2001 looked at 103 children aged six to eighteen years who had been diagnosed with earache. An herbal ear oil (made of garlic, mullein, calendula, and St. John's wort) was compared to an anesthetic drug ear drop. The herbal ear oil was as effective as the drug.[23]

Headache

Willow bark (*Salix alba* and other species) is nature's aspirin for headache and joint pain. Willow is a traditional pain reliever that still lives up to its reputation. Willow contains salicin and other related salicylates, which are the herbal forerunners of aspirin.[24] Salicylates such as those in willow, relieve pain, lower fever, and diminish inflammation. According to *The American Herbal Pharmacopoeia*, "in modern herbal therapy, willow is predominantly used as an anti-inflammatory for symptomatic relief of gouty arthritis and as an analgesic for mild neuralgic pains, toothaches and headaches."

Aspirin thins the blood, but willow bark does not, so don't use it for heart disease.[25] On the other hand, it won't cause the bleeding problems common with aspirin. Patients don't experience the typical digestive disturbances of aspirin when using willow.

There are no special warnings for using willow. Use a tea brewed from up to 1 ounce of the raw herb per day or an extract containing 240 milligrams total salicin per day. Willow can be used for as long as necessary.

Hemorrhoids

Beet root is the time-honored treatment for hemorrhoids around the globe. It stimulates the liver to produce more bile, promoting circulation through the liver and reducing pressure on the portal vein, the site of hemorrhoids (which is actually a varicose vein in the rectum). Carrot is milder, but will also work. Just eat a very large quantity of beet root or beet greens until the pain and itching lessen. Continue until you get complete relief.

Hemorrhoids respond particularly well to turmeric. Use up to 4 tablespoons per day of the bulk powder until the pain is gone. Turmeric is an astringent that shrinks swollen tissue. It can be used both orally and applied topically as a paste. Turmeric-based hemorrhoid creams are widely available in Asia. The paste is bright yellow, however, so remember that you may end up being yellow where you won't want to be yellow! (Only temporarily, though.)

Menstrual Cramps

Cinnamon bark excels in treating menstrual cramps. Many American women have found it to be a dramatic remedy, often giving relief on the first try, after years of monthly pain.

Like dong quai, cinnamon is a warming herb, which in Chinese terms means that it "warms the middle and disperses cold." This quality makes it a very good choice to promote menstruation. Since cinnamon enhances circulation to the uterus, the warm relaxing blood can relieve the cramps. As you would imagine, cinnamon is often used together with dong quai for this symptom. Cinnamon is a pungent, sweet, and hot yang tonic. The classic patient who can use cinnamon is cold, dry, and frail, and often has osteoarthritis, asthma, and digestive problems.

Since cinnamon is common as a culinary herb, it is necessary to be a selective shopper to get good quality. You will find medicinal-quality cinnamon in your health food store or Chinese herb pharmacy.

Nausea

Ginger's effect on motion sickness and nausea has been thoroughly proven, so it's not surprising that European practitioners use ginger as a tea for indigestion. It reduces spasm, absorbs and neutralizes toxins in the gastrointestinal tract, and increases the secretion of digestive juices, including bile and saliva.[26] Ginger contains ingredients that soothe the gut and aid digestion by increasing peristalsis that moves food through the intestine.

Sunburn

The flowering tops of St. John's wort (*Hypericum perforatum*) are nature's medicine for sunburn and nerve injury. This remedy has become the all-time phenomenon of the natural healing world. Expanding from anonymity to a household name in a few short years, it has become a mainstay in the self-care armamentarium. The flowers of this herb are commonly used for mild to moderate depression. Hypericum is an ancient medicine, however, and has been used in Europe for hundreds of years. Clinically, European and North American herbalists use the herb to benefit mild painful conditions, including arthritis, neuralgia, sciatica, and muscle inflammation.[27]

St. John's wort may be more known in Europe as an external remedy, which is the form in which it really excels. It is one of the most popular European remedies, used as an ointment for wounds, muscle pain, bruises, varicose veins, and burns.[28] St. John's wort flowers, which are yellow, contain red pigments, so the oil is a beautiful deep red color. Hypericum is especially therapeutic for sunburn, which is ironic, considering the photosensitivity it causes.

Some experts recommend not using hypericum concurrently with pharmaceutical antidepressants. The typical dose is 2 to 5 grams of raw herb, 10 to 15 milliliters of tincture, or 900 milligrams of standardized extract (0.3 percent hypericin), per day.

Natural medicine provides a treasure trove of home remedies. Most people on the planet treat any and all of their daily aches, pains, sniffles, bumps, and bruises with home-grown medicine. If you are aware of your diet choices, you can avoid a good share of these maladies. And if they do grab you, you can get a lot of mileage out of dietary adjustments.

When simple dietary adjustments don't pack the punch required to remedy your ills, move up to concentrated food remedies. For example, a glass of celery juice can halt a hay fever attack in its tracks! Herbal medicine is the next step. You should leave the heavy hitters to the professionals, but you can feel safe and secure using a dozen or so home remedies, like the rest of the world does. If you can master ten or twelve simple, easy-to-use natural medicines and have them available for home crises, you can stave off 90 percent of daily discomforts, from constipation to sunburn. Of course, you would have learned all about them from Grandma had you grown up in a traditional culture, but you can master them today with just a little effort and experimentation.

14

Specific Diseases and Treatments

According to Dr. Susan Lark, approximately 6 to 8 percent of us are naturally high-alkaline producers. These folks are natural peak performers. They have excellent lung capacity. Their digestive systems function well. They have strong skeletons with large reserves of alkaline minerals in their bones. Believe it or not, they thrive on stress, can eat the standard American diet with less ill effects, require hard endurance exercise, and rarely get ill. To top it off, they also age more slowly. Their natural edge on the rest of us shows up in extraordinary success. Where do I sign up?

Those are the fortunate few. But even if you didn't start with a naturally high-alkaline metabolism, you can regain the pH balance in your body. Would you like to regain your physical stamina, your optimism, and your ability to be sociable? To say nothing about tolerating the stresses of career and family. When you're in pH balance, you can again think clearly. You resist disease. Even if illness and injury should strike, you recover rapidly.

It just takes some study and determination to change the way you always do things.

Not Just Food, Minerals, and Herbs

Everything we do in our lives affects our pH balance one way or the other. Diet is almost always the most important factor because it's the area where most Americans have done the worst for the longest. In addition, it's the area that can have the most impact the fastest. It's also the area that Americans can relate to. Americans are used to hearing about different diets and about adjusting the diet for health. Most have tried a few changes. So they might be willing to be more experimental in this area than with some technique that is less familiar.

But that doesn't mean that there are not other excellent therapies that will benefit pH balance.

Siri Atma Singh Khalsa, M.D., who practices at Reality Health Center, in Española, New Mexico, uses the understanding of pH to help assess natural healing interventions in therapeutic situations. Dr. Khalsa is also a yoga teacher. In addition to dietary and herbal recommendations for adjusting pH, he likes to prescribe breathing techniques. He told me that he especially likes a kundalini yoga technique called "breath of fire." This rapid diaphragmatic breath flushes excess carbon dioxide from the blood, balancing the body by diminishing the store of carbonic acid.

Even though exercise causes calories to be burned, producing acids, and muscle movement produces lactic acid, it's still better to do it than not. (No score here for the couch potato, sorry.)

Yoga is a system designed from the ground up to restore and maintain health. I've been practicing and teaching yoga for thirty years. It can work miracles for health. As the sister science of Ayurveda, it comes from the same origins and shares the same philosophy.

The Senior Years

As we age, many factors conspire to pull our pH out of balance.

Dr. Roberta Lee calls the kidney "the great regulator." As normal kidney function decreases with age, metabolic acidosis gradually increases. This causes valuable calcium, often already in short supply, and needed for buffering and bone strength, to slip away in the urine.

The aging stomach begins to produce less acid, further retarding mineral absorption and protein digestion. To add to this problem, many seniors do not consume enough protein. The pH can begin to creep toward the alkaline side. This is catabolic: It causes accelerated tissue destruction and loss, weakening a body that is perhaps already frail. Dr. Brown says it is not uncommon to see a pH of 8.0 or more in elderly persons. Use a kit to measure pH and compensate by upping protein sources. Dr.

Brown says that elders may require one to two servings of flesh food each day to maintain bone and protein reserves. Other colleagues think it can be done with nonmeat proteins, even in the senior years.

Treatment of Individual Diseases

Body balancing is important to our general health. Using the techniques in this book, we can stay healthy. But what if something has already gone wrong? Can we treat it with body-balancing methods? Without reservation, the answer is yes. Specific tissues have their own characteristic healthy pH. We can measure the acidity of some tissues, apply treatment, and gauge the results.

With some other conditions, the symptoms are so distinctive that we can deduce the pH problem from the body's presentation, apply treatment based on our best guesswork, and assess the result according to the experience of change we get with the body. One thing is for sure: Natural methods work. Body chemistry is so basic that it influences every disease to which the body can succumb. In this section, we will look at a small collection of common examples.

Acne and Dermatitis

You spend a lifetime living in your skin and a good chunk of your paycheck induging it. Most important, it's the barrier between you and the hostile world outside you. Clearly, it's critically important to keep your skin strong and healthy.

"Dermatitis" is a broad term for a wide assortment of skin disorders. The word actually means "inflammation of the skin." True dermatitis involves a superficial inflammation, with blisters when acute, as well as redness, swelling, oozing, crusting, scaling, and usually itching. As a disease category, dermatitis is divided into two main groups. "Endogenous" conditions arise from problems in the body itself and include "atopic dermatitis," which is caused by an unknown, usually hereditary, allergic process. "Exogenous" conditions result from outside sources and include "contact dermatitis," such as poison oak reactions.

Health practitioners use many terms to describe various combinations of these common skin symptoms. "Eczema" is synonymous with dermatitis. Authorities do not generally agree about any distinction between these conditions. "Psoriasis" is characterized by dry scaly patches, called "plaques." Acne, which can begin even in midlife, includes especially the inflammation of the hair follicles and sebaceous glands.

Adults with the usual mishmash of these symptoms may receive a diagnosis of any of these disease names. From the natural healing point of view, though, this whole process is the final manifestation of the same underlying situation, and we can conveniently label all these conditions as "inflammatory skin disease."

Acne, or what could be called inflammatory skin disease, is the absolute classic acid, hot, inflamed, toxic, pitta condition. Body-balancing and pH therapies work beautifully.

Detoxification is the key. Natural healing practitioners the world over understand that inflammatory skin disease is fundamentally a problem of accumulated waste material in the body. These undesirable wastes, which come from outside the body (pesticides, pollution) or inside the body (accumulated cellular wastes), irritate the skin and cause the persistent inflammation. In fact, in Ayurveda, the name for this disorder translates as "that which comes out from the inner part to the outer part."

Herbal medicine focuses on reducing inflammation in the skin, healing the tissue of the skin if necessary, and eliminating the source of the irritating toxins through the liver, kidneys, and large intestine. (For help with the dietary management of acne, see "Acne and Diet" below.)

Acne and Diet

In the case of acne, Americans are right in looking to the diet for assistance in managing the condition. Foods to favor in your diet include the following:

Foods to avoid include the following:

Asparagus	Chard
Avocado	Chickpeas
Barley	Cilantro
Basil	Collard
Beets	Cucumber
Broccoli	Dandelion greens
Burdock	Fig
Carrots	Millet

Mung beans	Spinach
Parsley	Walnut
Raisin	Whole rice
Shiitake mushrooms	

Alcohol	Fried or oily food
Cheese	Saturated or hydrogenated fat
Chocolate	Processed food
Citrus	Red meat
Coffee	Sugar
Eggs	Tomatoes

In addition, to prevent or control acne, avoid high-protein diets.

After you begin to apply pH-balancing principles and the skin begins to settle down, it's time to heal the underlying structure of the tissue. Gotu kola (*Centella asiatica*) is a well-known remedy in Ayurvedic medicine that is just beginning to be available here. A famous herb in India, it's the most spectacular herb I've ever seen in treating damage, not only to skin, but to all types of connective tissue.

This herb has been around the fringes of European herbalism for many years. In fact, it was used in France in the 1880s. The active substances in gotu kola are thought to be triterpenes (steroidlike compounds), which have a balancing effect on connective tissues. These triterpenes improve the function and integrity of the collagen matrix and support the "ground substance," the basic "glue" that holds the cells of our bodies together.

Known for centuries in Asia for its treatment of leprosy, gotu kola heals a host of corrupt skin conditions, including wounds, cellulite, varicose veins, and dermatitis. It stimulates the growth of hair and nails, increases blood supply to connective tissue, enhances the formation of structural constituents in connective tissue, promotes the tensile integrity of the skin, and increases protein growth (keratinization) in the skin.

These qualities give gotu kola the ability to actually heal and grow new skin, gently closing and repairing even long-standing, painful lesions and skin ulcers. The herb also heals scars. Several studies have shown impressive results in the treatment of even dramatically scarred skin.

An impressive study of gotu kola in the treatment of scleroderma, an extreme inflammatory skin disease characterized by poor wound healing and scar formation, was done twenty-five years ago in Europe. Even at a very conservative dose, gotu kola was effective in 85 percent of the patients.[1]

Arthritis

I can hardly imagine anything more wretched than the prospect of facing the rest of life with increasing daily pain, leading eventually to a slow slide into disability. But millions of osteoarthritis sufferers are facing just that future.

The term "arthritis" literally means "joint inflammation," but it is commonly used to denote a diverse collection of more than 100 rheumatic diseases that cause pain, stiffness, and swelling in joints and may also affect other parts of the body, primarily other connective tissue structures. These arthritis diseases afflict nearly 43 million Americans. Arthritis is the most common cause of disability in people sixty-five and older.

Osteoarthritis (OA), or degenerative joint disease (DJG), is the most common form of joint disease. The disease increases in prevalence with age. About 5 percent of Americans are affected with hip or knee osteoarthritis, while 9.5 percent of adults over sixty-two have osteoarthritis of the knee. Because of its high rate of occurrence and associated pain and dysfunction, osteoarthritis accounts for much of the disability in the lower extremities in the elderly. Osteoarthritis accounts for more than 70 percent of total hip and knee replacements.

OA is typified by erosion of joint cartilage. In an aging body, the water composition of cartilage increases while the protein composition degenerates, causing the cartilage to form tiny crevasses. Over time, cartilage surfaces fray, wear, ulcerate, and in extreme cases, wear down completely, leaving the joint to chafe bone-on-bone, causing pain and limiting joint mobility. Bony spurs may form at joint edges.

In the long run, OA causes joint pain, loss of function, reduced joint motion, and deformity. OA most often affects the knees, hips, spine, and hands, and sometimes other joints. Ultimately, disability may result from disease in the spine, knees, or hips.

Previously, OA was thought to be a progressive, degenerative disor-

der and was widely known as "wear-and-tear arthritis."
that everyone, if they lived long enough, would fall prey
known, however, that the disease can be arrested or rev
idence has changed the thinking about the disease progress or OA. we
now know that the joint cartilage of patients with OA is highly metabolically active. The damaged cartilage tissue actually tries to remodel
and repair itself. Though once thought to be impossible, arresting or reversing the disease occurs spontaneously in some OA patients.

Conventional medicine considers arthritis to be incurable but man-
ageable. Most treatment programs include a medication, exercise, rest,
heat and cold therapies, joint protection techniques, and sometimes
surgery.

Pharmacological treatments for all forms of arthritis are fairly similar
and include nonsteroidal anti-inflammatory drugs (NSAIDs), such as
ibuprofen and naproxen, and painkillers, including salicylates such as ac-
etaminophen and aspirin. These drugs effectively decrease joint pain and
increase mobility.

Drugs can relieve symptoms, but they are far from perfect. NSAIDs,
especially, cause serious side effects, including ulcers and liver and kidney failure. In fact, more than 100,000 patients are hospitalized and
16,500 die each year in the United States from NSAID-related gastrointestinal problems. It's because of these adverse effects that sufferers of
arthritis are turning to alternative and nutritional therapy.

Neither of these types of medications cures the underlying cause of
the disease. Evidence suggests, in fact, in both animals and humans, that
NSAIDs may actually accelerate joint destruction. In addition, test-tube
studies indicate that some of these drugs adversely affect the protein metabolism of articular cartilage. NSAIDs suppress synthesis of proteoglycans (the slippery molecules in synovial fluid) by the cartilage cell
(chondrocyte). Animal studies further suggest that salicylate drugs may
accelerate cartilage damage in osteoarthritis. Since depletion of cartilage
matrix proteoglycans appears to be a major factor in the increased vul-
nerability of chondrocyte in degenerating cartilage, it looks like, despite
the symptomatic improvement that these drugs produce, they don't slow
the progression of the disease, and they probably accelerate cartilage degeneration.

Arthritis pain is caused by several factors. Inflammation is the process
that causes the redness and swelling in joints. Damage to joint tissues results from the disease process or from stress, injury, or pressure on the

,oints. Fatigue, which can make your pain seem worse and more difficult to tolerate, results from the disease process. Depression and stress result from the limited movement and not being able to participate in enjoyable activities any longer. Each facet of joint pain must be approached in a distinctive and appropriate way. One way to reduce pain is to build a life around wellness, not pain or sickness.

From the natural therapy point of view, the energy of OA is cold and dry. OA is a vata disease that occurs in "hypometabolic" people—that is, people with low body temperature and slow metabolic rate. These bodies have difficulty retaining fluids in the tissues, so there is a general lack of lubrication, including of the joint surfaces. The overall result is stiffness and pain.

Following this reasoning, the overall treatment strategy for OA is to warm the tissues, increase mobility, and enhance moisture and lubrication throughout the body. A comprehensive program of bodywork, diet, and herbal medicine can be very effective.

California poppy (*Eschscholtzia californica*) is nature's remedy for arthritis. This delightful garden plant is actually powerful medicine. Originally used by Native Americans, it is distantly related to opium poppies and contains isoquinoline alkaloids, which are known to have pain-relieving properties. This American herb has become a popular pain medicine in Europe.[2] *The Complete German Commission E Monographs* lists it as an antispasmodic and sedative. The aerial parts (leaf, flower, and stem) are the medicinal parts.

California poppy is relaxing, so it works well in cases of pain with anxiety and insomnia. A 1991 animal study from France showed a definite anti-anxiety effect. Higher doses were sedative.[3] A key alkaloid (chelerthyrine) was shown to inhibit a body protein (kinase C) that contributes to persistent pain.[4,5]

A German study showed that an extract of the plant had analgesic properties in the test tube.[6]

Since California poppy is relaxing and promotes sleep, don't take it while driving, and exceed the recommended dose only with caution. Increase the dose gradually until you are familiar with the pain-relieving and sedative effects. As tea, a typical dose is 3 to 5 teaspoons of chopped dry herb, brewed, taken when necessary. As a tincture, start with 5 milliliters when necessary and adjust for pain.

Asthma

Asthma involves a restriction in breathing. More correctly called "reactive airway disease," it can involve spasm of the airway, inflammation of the tracheal tissues, or both. Some asthma—so-called wet asthma—includes copious respiratory mucus. Many cases of asthma include a trigger, such as exposure to cold air or an allergic reaction, that starts the constrictive episode.

Dr. Tillotson reminds us that "asthma patients, in particular, tend to be overalkaline." Carefully evaluate your pH situation with one of the methods we have discussed and adjust, if necessary, in the proper direction.

Basil helps shortness of breath and bronchiospasm in asthma.[7] Garlic is used in some cases of asthma in Ayurveda.

Schisandra (*Schisandra chinensis*) is an East Asian woody vine in the magnolia family. Winding around the trunks of trees and covering the branches, the vine produces small red berries that grow in clusters. In the fall, the berries are harvested and dried to make the medicinal herb.

The Chinese name for this herb is *wu wei tze*, or "five-flavor berry," indicating that the fruit contains all five flavors of the Chinese herbal pharmacy. Herbs with this taste profile are rare, and this detail predicts schisandra's use in a wide variety of conditions. Schisandra is mostly sour, though, and most definitely astringent.

Chinese medicine considers schisandra specific for asthma. The astringent qualities of the berry make it ideal for what the Chinese call "preserving the essence"—keeping leaking fluids retained where they belong. Used predominantly for the lungs and kidneys to arrest mucous discharges, this ability marks schisandra for bed-wetting, urinary incontinence, postnasal drip, and spermatorrhea, the involuntary loss of semen. In my experience as a clinical herbalist, this remedy is especially effective for night sweats.

Schisandra berries actually taste pretty good, so they can be taken as a tea or even cooked into food, such as soup broth. This herb is quite mild and foodlike, so feel free to use as much as you care. Use a high dose acutely, then a small daily dose for maintenance. The TCM dose for acute conditions is 10 grams per day in food or tea. The maintenance dose is 1 to 2 grams per day. Remember that the effects are slow and gradual, and extend over a period of years.

Canker Sores

Commonly called "canker sores," but more correctly termed aphthous ulcers, these mouth ulcers can be supremely painful. Canker sores are inflamed areas in the mucous membranes of the mouth. As the spot becomes more involved, the local mucous tissue breaks down. Canker sores are invariably a sign of excess acidity in the mouth, and in the body in general. Do not confuse these painful mouth ulcers with cold sores, which are caused by a virus in the herpes family.

Jonathan Wright, M.D., of Kent, Washington, says that canker sores are virtually always linked to food allergies and nutritional deficiencies, particularly of iron, vitamin B_{12}, and folic acid. He also suggests using high oral doses of acidophilus and an acidophilus mouth rinse.[8]

Since mouth ulcers stem from a breakdown in tissue structure, the herb gotu kola can be quite effective. Gotu kola is widely known to heal wounds and promote connective tissue growth. The daily dose is 1 ounce of herb, brewed as tea, or a smaller dose, to tolerance, in capsules.

Other rinses that can help include alum, milk of magnesia, and cinchona bark. Many people benefit from retaining a chewable tablet of alkaline calcium in the mouth as long as possible. Noted natural physician Hakim Chishti suggests the powder of myrrh gum applied directly to the ulcer.

Probably the most outstanding herbal remedy for mouth sores is licorice root, a potent anti-inflammatory and tissue healer. Put a pinch of powder on the sore or suck on a lozenge made from DGL.

Cold and Flu

Cold and flu (short for "influenza") are viral diseases that affect the respiratory tract. Influenza is a stronger bug, although it produces basically the same symptoms. Body chemistry that is out of balance can weaken the immune system, as we have seen. Now you have no need to suffer and no need to use drugs to get a good night's sleep while you are fighting that pesky cough. Natural medicine can help you stay comfortable, even when the bug has bitten you.

Osha root (*Ligusticum porteri*) and its cousins are found growing in the high altitudes in the southwest and Rocky Mountain states. This herb is a traditional Native American remedy for respiratory infections. Herbalists often recommended osha root for use at the first sign of a respiratory infection. It is used as a cough suppressant and expectorant, garnering it the common name "Colorado cough root." It's clear that the herb contains anti-inflammatory ingredients.[9] A 1994 Chinese study showed benefit for reducing respiratory inflammation, reducing bronchial spasm, and improving lung function.[10]

Research from China also indicates that Szechuan lovage root can relax smooth muscle tissue and inhibit the growth of various bacteria.[11]

Ever wonder why all cough syrups are cherry flavored? Wild cherry bark (*Prunus serotina*), a North American herb, was the absolute standby for coughs in times past. The bark has a pleasant cherry taste when prepared as a medicine. The medicine contains cyanogenic glycosides, especially prunasin. These glycosides, metabolized in the body, act to suppress spasms in the smooth muscles lining the bronchioles, providing cough relief. Theoretically, extremely large doses of wild cherry pose a risk of cyanide poisoning. This has not been observed in clinical practice, though, so it is agreed that cherry is a very safe herbal remedy.

The slippery elm tree (*Ulmus rubra*) is native to North America. Native Americans made canoes, baskets, and other household goods from the tree and its bark. Slippery elm, a soothing, slimy herb, was used internally for sore throats and diarrhea. As a poultice, it was a useful remedy for skin conditions.

Slippery elm bark is another mucilage-containing, throat-soothing medicine. The FDA has deemed the herb a safe, effective cough soother.[12]

Constipation

Regular, bulky, and soft bowel movements are fundamental to good health. But an awful lot of Americans are constipated. Constipation is medically defined as passing stools less than three times a week or in low quantity, but natural healing proponents say that a bowel movement for each meal is fine and that at least one per day is essential. Any less might be caused by one of the three critical factors. You may become constipated if the stool is too dry or has too little fiber content. If the large intestine has lost its zip and peristalsis has slowed, there could be a bit of a bowel backup.

Psyllium seed, a common bulk fiber laxative, balances bowel function and relieves pain in irritable bowels.[13] Psyllium's capacity to absorb fluids means that it is useful for treating diarrhea. As it travels through the gut, the mucilage in psyllium is soothing, which may relieve cramping. An

English study revealed that constipation significantly improved in patients taking psyllium. A total of 82 percent of the subjects had irritable bowel symptom relief.[14] A study to determine the optimum dose recommended 20 grams per day.[15]

Proper moisture content is critical for good elimination. Including what we drink and digestive secretions, about five gallons of fluid is dumped into the large intestine every day. Most of this has to be reabsorbed or we would quickly become dehydrated. Mucilages are herbs that create a healing slime that coats and soothes the gut wall and keeps the stool moist and slippery enough to exit smoothly. These include marshmallow root (*Althea officinalis*), slippery elm bark (*Ulmus spp.*), and mullein leaf (*Verbascum spp.*). Marshmallow is used for inflammation of the stomach membranes.[16] To use marshmallow or slippery elm, take 1 tablespoon of powdered bulk herb per meal (stirred into a bite of food, such as applesauce, if desired).

Osmotic laxatives, including the natural mineral magnesium, draw moisture into the bowel and soften stool. Most people can tolerate up to about 1,200 milligrams of magnesium per day.

Gallstones

A gallbladder attack is a horrible experience. Usually the patient has just finished a nice, filling meal, probably high in fat, and is relaxing, lying down. Then the wrenching pain starts. Many people who have gone through this say that it's the worst pain they have ever felt, comparable to childbirth. Then the nausea and sweating begin. After seemingly endless hours of this, the symptoms eventually subside. Never wanting to feel even a fraction of that again, the patient runs to the doctor. Usually the gallbladder is removed as a matter of course. Avoiding this scenario at any cost becomes the order of business. You can see why early diagnosis is so essential.

Gallstones are lumps of solid matter that form in the interior space of the gallbladder or in the common bile duct. Cholesterol gallstones are composed mainly of cholesterol, which is made in the liver. Excess cholesterol is removed from the blood by the liver and is then secreted into bile. When bile contains abundant cholesterol, small crystals form, finally settling at the bottom of the gallbladder. These cholesterol crystals fuse together in the gallbladder to form stones. This type of gallstone accounts for nearly 80 percent of all cases of gallstones in the United States.

Herbalists have a large collection of potent techniques with which to treat gallbladder disease. These remedies usually are quite successful. However, they tend to be slow, even in the best of circumstances. Often, by the time a person realizes that he or she even has gallstones, the symptoms have become quite uncomfortable. At that stage, many people can no longer bear the discomfort and choose to follow through with surgery to remove the gallbladder. So, early diagnosis is essential. Clinically, I have not had a single client who failed to improve and required subsequent surgery.

Gallbladder treatment uses the following types of herbs:

- Anti-inflammatory herbs, to reduce swelling.
- Anti-spasmodics, to reduce constriction.
- Hepatics, to generally benefit the liver.
- Immune enhancers, to fight chronic infection.
- Nervines, to ease pain and stress.
- Cholagogues, to thin the bile and increase bile production. (Note that these must be used with caution, as they may increase contractions.)

The following cholagogues are the first line of attack. Remember, they must be used carefully. As a general rule, cholagogues tend to be nauseating and to cause loose stool. Since constipation is characteristic of this condition, however, this can be a benefit. In fact, many of these cholagogues are listed as purgatives. Inducing bile flow is a typical way of promoting bowel action. Also, causing an unwanted sudden contraction of the gallbladder may cause, at the least, an acute attack and, at the worst, may lodge a stone in the duct, which causes the patient to end up in the hospital.

Stone root (*Collinsonia canadensis*) is one of my personal favorites for this condition. Although not typically listed in materia medica as a cholagogue, this herb, which I learned about from old-time naturopathic physicians years ago, has stood the test of time. Usually considered an herb for hemorrhoids, it is often cited as working on the veins as an astringent. My teachers claimed that it works on the liver to enhance bile flow, thus treating hemorrhoids through release of pressure on the portal vein. Be that as it may, it is effective for gallbladder disease. Of all the herbs I have used, this one has consistently produced the most results for chronic conditions, with intermittent acute attacks.

The dose in capsules is 500 to 5,000 milligrams per day, depending on bowel tolerance, in divided, incrementally increasing doses, taken with food. Watch carefully for queasiness, and adjust the dose increment.

The simple dandelion root (*Taraxacum officinale*) is stalwart medicine. Although most of us fight this bright yellow flower as a common lawn pest, herbalists the world over have held dandelion in high regard for centuries. In fact, dandelion is a major herb in at least three ancient herbal traditions: Western, Chinese, and Ayurveda. This herb is bitter and cold, and due to its high mineral content, a bit salty, making it effective for conditions of "damp heat," in Chinese herbal parlance—conditions such as jaundice.

Dandelion contains bitter glycosides, the bitter resin taraxacerin, phytosterols (including sitosterol), tannins, triterpenes, a wide variety of minerals, notably potassium and calcium, and several vitamins, including A and C.

Dandelion root is higher in nutrient content than many other vegetables. For example, carrot has 11,000 international units of vitamin A, a necessary liver nutrient, per 100 grams. Dandelion, on the other hand, has a whopping 14,000 international units.[17]

Human and animal studies show that dandelion increases bile flow, benefiting liver congestion, bile duct inflammation, and gallstones.

Dandelion acts in two ways to increase bile flow. It causes the liver to produce more bile to send to the gallbladder (choleretic effect), and it acts directly on the gallbladder, causing it to contract and release stored bile (cholagogue effect).

Drs. Pizzorno and Murray call dandelion one of the finest remedies for the "sluggish, congested, toxic liver." Although the leaf is also medicinal, acting as a powerful diuretic, which of course also detoxifies through the kidneys, the root is the noted liver cleanser.

Dandelion root can be taken as tea, tincture, or capsules. A good dose is 3,000 milligrams per day. Roasted dandelion root is brewed as a delicious coffee substitute.

Used mainly as an exotic vegetable, globe artichoke (Cynara scolymus) is a thistlelike plant in the daisy family. However, this plant is used herbally as an excellent detoxifier of the liver and gallbladder. In Europe, artichoke therapy is so important that an entire segment of phytomedicine is called "cynotherapy."

Artichoke contains a sesquiterpene lactone called cynaropicrin, which accounts for its characteristic bitter taste. Another substance more recently isolated called cynarin promotes bile flow and has antitoxic liver functions similar to another well-known liver detoxifying herb, milk thistle. Artichoke promotes liver regeneration and brings blood to the liver. It also reduces blood fats, like cholesterol, by a mechanism similar to niacin, and effectively treats gallstones. Its fat-lowering effects make it valuable in treating obesity. One study showed a significant reduction in elevated cholesterol (12.2 percent) and triglyceride (5.7 percent) levels with artichoke extract. These patients also lost body weight.[18]

Artichoke leaf would normally be consumed as a vegetable, but the raw globe can also be juiced. Artichoke extract, made from the whole plant, is available as a dietary supplement.

Another member of the daisy family, burdock root (*Arctium lappa*), a native of Eurasia, is now firmly established in North America. The genus name, *Arctium*, is from the Greek *arktos*, meaning "bear," a reference to its rough burrs. The species, *lappa*, comes from "to seize," a similar reference.

Burdock is rich in flavonoids, lignans, and bitter glycosides. It has an inulin content of up to 45 percent, making it valuable in treating diabetes. The high levels of lignans and inulin have demonstrated anti-inflammatory activities, explaining its use in damp heat ("fire toxins" in Chinese medicine) conditions such as acute laryngitis and skin inflammation.

Burdock has a long history of use as a detoxifier in skin conditions. It is said to be a "general alterative"—that is, it influences the skin, kidneys, and mucous and serous membranes, to remove accumulated waste products. It is specific for eruptions on the head, face, and neck, and for acute irritable and inflammatory conditions.[19] It could be used for eczema, psoriasis, boils, and similar skin toxicity conditions.

The root is cultivated as a food in Japan, where it is called *gobo*. Resembling a long brown carrot, it can be prepared in any way you might enjoy a carrot, such as juiced or steamed. Try steaming a half-and-half mixture of carrot and burdock slices, serving them with dill or a light sauce. Since burdock is more powerful as a cleanser than carrot, it is also practical to prepare a tea from the chopped dried root. The dose would be .25 ounce of the dried herb, brewed, per day. The equivalent in capsules could also be used.

Turmeric is one of my favorite herbs. A very safe herb, it is used in food. In fact, it gives the yellow color to curry powders. A very broad-spectrum herb, its uses are numerous. This herb is widely used in Ayurveda as a liver detoxifier. The active compounds, called curcuminoids, are comparable to the active ingredients in licorice and milk thistle seed.

Like the herbs discussed above, turmeric increases bile flow and is useful in jaundice. Studies show that increases in liver inflammation, measured by blood tests, are prevented by turmeric.[20] Turmeric is a powerful antioxidant, comparable in effect to vitamins E and C.[21] It also reduces formation of many toxins produced from animal fat in the diet, suppressing cancer and inflammation.

Use up to 4 tablespoons of turmeric powder per day in food, stirred into water as a drink, or in capsules.

Magnesium may be of value at bowel-tolerance doses, generally around 1,600 milligrams per day, as it moisturizes and loosens the stool.

Menthol and related terpenes (menthone, pinene, bornoel, cineole, and camphene) have shown promise for gallstone treatment. They can be used for extended periods, up to several years. Terpenes reduce bile cholesterol levels, while also increasing bile acid and lecithin levels in the biliary system. I have had very good clinical success in reversing gallstone symptoms in cases diagnosed by ultrasound using peppermint powder in capsules, oral peppermint oil, and encapsulated camphor. In particular, peppermint is very effective for the aggravating chronic burping that often accompanies this syndrome.

Charcoal capsules can be beneficial for the gas that accompanies gallbladder disease. Use at the dose that produces the greatest relief.

Calcium (in carbonate form), taken with a meal, sometimes prevents symptoms from symptom-prone foods. Calcium has also been shown to be protective for the stones, as it binds secondary bile acids in the colon, allowing them to be excreted. Digestive enzymes can be likewise effective.

Vitamin C at doses of 2,000 milligrams per day positively effects the composition of bile, thus reducing cholesterol-based stones. Diets deficient in vitamin E provoke gallstones, and vitamin E supplementation reduces the tendency of the bile to form cholesterol stones. The amino acid taurine conjugates bile acids and increases bile flow and excretion.

Gastritis and Ulcer

The entire digestive tract is lined with mucous membrane. The tissue is pretty much the same from one end to the other. If the tissue becomes inflamed, or if the integrity of the tissue structure breaks down, the powerful digestive juices in the digestive tube can irritate or damage the tissue. Inflammation in the gut is named for the area that is stricken. If it's in the stomach, it's called gastritis; if it's in the ileum, ileitis; the colon, colitis; and so on. If the upper layer of mucus thins out and the underlying tissue layers begin to break down, an ulcer results. Ulcerations can occur anywhere along the length of the tract, although it's more common to refer to an ulcer in the stomach (peptic ulcer) or the small intestine (duodenal ulcer).

Chanchal Cabrera sees a lot of gastritis (heartburn) and esophagitis in her practice in Ashland, Oregon. She sees a lot of cancer patients who have just undergone chemotherapy. The powerful cancer drugs damage the stomach lining cells and reduce gastric mucus flow. She uses slippery elm bark to coat and sooth the burning. Since this herb is rich in nutritive starches, it also supplies a little food value for these exhausted patients. Marshmallow root powder works almost as well. Meadowsweet is also an herb that reduces stomach inflammation and heals the lining, according to Chanchal.

Chanchal also uses N-acetyl glucosamine (NAG). This nutrient, an amino sugar, formed from a sugar and an amino acid, is directly involved in repairing the superficial mucous layers of the stomach.

Chanchal recommends consuming coating liquids such as milk, soy milk, nut milk, and yogurt, with small, frequent meals. Aloe vera inhibits gastric acid secretion and soothes the stomach lining.

Dr. Michael Murray suggests DGL, which is also effective for ulcers. DGL comes in chewable wafers that coat the digestive tract lining, cooling the burning.

Ultimately, the digestive tract is so similar along its length that the same remedies are likely to be effective for inflammation or ulcer just about anywhere in the gut.

Hay Fever and Allergy

Allergy is an inappropriately aggressive hypersensitivity reaction of the immune system to a specific substance. The offending substance (such as plant pollen, insect venom, drugs, or food) is called an allergen. In most people, exposure to the substance results in no symptoms. Affected people have a well-known complex of reactions, including tissue swelling, watery eyes, itching, skin redness, and respiratory mucus. If the allergen impacts the respiratory tract, it produces a condition called allergic rhinitis (inflammation of the nasal and sinus mucous membranes). Seasonal rhinitis, caused by specific seasonal tree, grass, or weed pollens, is sometimes called "hay fever." It is the most common of all allergic diseases in the United States, touching up to 10 percent of the adult population. Allergic rhinitis is not fatal, but the economic impact is substantial.

Nettle is a modern-day allergy miracle. Herbalists in clinical practice have been forming a consensus over the last decade that nettle leaf is effective for allergy symptoms. That has certainly been my experience. Although the scientific research remains preliminary, it continues to point to the anti-inflammatory properties of nettle.[22] One study showed that nettle produced an antiallergy effect.[23] Research seems to point to at least one of the active components being a bioflavonoid, although some authorities think it is characteristic polysaccharides and others believe it is lectins.

It's also known that nettles contain histamines, the same type of chemicals produced by the body in an allergic reaction. Another proposed mechanism for nettle is that the histamines in nettle attach to the histamine receptor sites in the body's cells, blocking your body's own histamines from attaching.

Whatever the final determination of the active ingredients, nettle loses its antiallergy power if it's not harvested and processed correctly. Look for a high-quality powdered product that has been freeze-dried or specially processed to retain the bioflavonoid. This special processing costs more; so don't be seduced by cheap imitations.

Many people take up to 3,000 milligrams of specially processed nettle leaf powder in capsules per day to relieve the temporary symptoms of hay fever and other allergic reactions, including animal allergy. Remember, this short-term use of nettle is not curative. Use nettle when you would otherwise use an antihistamine drug to stop your misery. Symptoms often begin to improve within fifteen minutes, and the effect typically lasts for about four hours.

This interest in nettle's anti-inflammatory properties is spawning a body of research investigating potential benefit for joint disease. Preliminary studies look good.[24] One 1997 study involving thirty-seven patients showed a 70 percent improvement in arthritis symptoms in just two weeks.[25]

Herpes Simplex

A cold sore is caused by a virus so contagious that it's spread simply through kissing. To make matters worse, it produces a sore that's more painful than a scrape or bruise, and uglier and more embarrassing than a big pimple. This revolting malady, apparently created just to ruin this weekend's big date, is in fact a viral disease. Cold sores are liquid-filled blisters that erupt around the lips and sometimes spread to the nose or chin. They are caused principally by herpes simplex virus type 1 (HSV-1), a common relative of the virus that causes chicken pox.

A related bug, the HSV-2 virus, causes genital herpes. Though quite similar in the symptoms they produce, these two varieties of virus are distinct. Oral infections (cold sores) are usually caused by type 1, while genital infections (venereal herpes) are products of type 2. Nonetheless, it is actually possible for either type to infect either tissue. Practically, these strains of virus are so similar that they respond to the same medicines, and for all practical purposes, they are treated with the same methods.

Contrary to popular belief, cold sores are not automatically the result of being cold or catching a cold, and can be just as unrelenting in summer as winter. Just about anything that insults the immune system can trigger an outbreak of cold sores, including a bout of cold or flu, emotional stress, fever, fatigue or overwork, hormonal changes including menstruation or pregnancy, local trauma to the mouth such as dental work or shaving, lack of sleep, excess alcohol or sugar, poor nutrition, and exposure to sun, wind, or cold weather. An outbreak lasts from six to ten days on average if left untreated. Sometimes the sores are accompanied by fever, swollen neck glands, and general body aches.

More than 60 percent of Americans have endured a cold sore at some time, and almost 25 percent suffer recurrent outbreaks. More than 90 percent of all adult oral herpes sufferers were infected as children, typically from an adult with a cold sore, when they were between the ages of six months and four years. The virus invades the moist membrane cells of the lips, throat, or mouth and initially causes no symptoms, with most cases being mild and unrecognized in the infant, often mistaken for teething or a cold. Though the child feels better in short order, the virus never leaves the body. The patient is at risk of a secondary flare-up at any time in later life.

Cold sores can be spread to other people by contact, including kissing and the sharing of objects such as toothbrushes, towels, knives, and forks. The disease can also be spread to other areas of your own body, so be vigilant about touching other membranes. Don't confuse cold sores with canker sores, correctly called aphthous ulcers, which are small ulcers that form on mucous membranes of the digestive tract, including the oral cavity. They are not caused by a virus.

Dr. Peshek believed that herpes lesions were caused by acid pH in the body.[26] Since he was a dentist, he got to observe many cases of oral herpes and drew conclusions about what was effective. He suggested a program based on alkalinizing the body. He used many remedies, including calcium lactate, at a dose of 1,000 milligrams of elemental calcium per day, between meals. He also reported success with a half teaspoon of sodium bicarbonate two hours before each meal. This small amount of bicarbonate will have a minor but noticeable effect on blood pH, according to Dr. Peshek.

For herpes, Dr. Peshek also recommended the amino acid methionine at 500 milligrams per day, in divided doses, and vitamin E at 40 international units per day. The Peshek program also included essential fatty acids, acidophilus, vitamin B-complex, and the alkalinizing mineral zinc.

My secret weapon for herpes of all types is the Chinese herb platycodon root. Also called balloon flower root, platycodon is a cooling antiviral herb. Use 12 grams per day, in capsules, for an acute episode, and 1 to 2 grams per day long term to control outbreaks.

Polyphenols are chemicals that form a large group of very active compounds in herbal medicines. They are anti-inflammatory, antiviral, immune enhancing, and astringent—just the qualities we look for in treating a blistering viral disease. In viral infections, polyphenol substances seem to latch on to the body's cellular virus receptor sites, taking up the space and prohibiting the virus from attaching to the cell, short-circuiting the bug's ability to cause infection. Popular herbs that are high in polyphenol content are turmeric root, bilberry fruit, and ginkgo leaf.

Lemon balm (*Melissa officinalis*), also known as melissa, is probably the most well-respected herbal treatment for cold sores in use in this country today. Melissa is a European herb, and most of the research on this effective plant comes from there. Although the action of melissa is not completely explained, it appears that the antiviral effects are the result of the high content of polyphenols in the leaf. Lemon balm is a member of the mint family, so it is a pleasant herb to work with, with a delicious taste and smell. Melissa provides effective pain relief within eight hours and performs as well as acyclovir cream, the leading drug for oral herpes. A highly potent (concentrated seventy times) melissa extract is made into an ointment. Traditionally, essential oil of melissa at a 1 percent concentration has been used in the cream. Melissa ointments are widely available as commercial preparations from the herb store. Apply the salve directly to the blister.

If you're more of a do-it-yourselfer, brew lemon balm as tea, drink the tea for its antiviral effect, squeeze out the dregs, and apply the moist dregs as a mush directly to the sore, allowing the mass to stay put for an hour or two. Then again, you can soak cotton gauze in the tea itself and apply it to the blister.

Other, more familiar mints also have general antiviral properties and will probably work just about as well as melissa. Mints are all rich sources of antiviral components, including caffeic acid, quercitin, tannic acid, and thymol. To keep viruses at bay, Dr. Duke advocates drinking several strongly brewed cups of a tea made from an assortment of good-tasting mints—hyssop, lemon balm, oregano, rosemary, sage, self-heal, and thyme.

Capsaicin, the active compound in cayenne and other chilies, is a potent antiviral. This herb is one of my personal favorites for healing cold sores and, in fact, genital herpes. It works fast, it's effective, the dose is reasonable, it's affordable, and it's available. Dr. Duke also proposes red chili pepper for its scientifically proven ability to prevent outbreaks of herpes. Take cayenne internally to treat the virus. Sprinkle it on your food, if you dare, or take it in a capsule to avoid the sting. This herb is very spicy, so take it with a meal. Start with a very small dose, say, a half capsule, to assess your comfort level. Gradually increase the dose until you get relief from the pain of the blister, which typically occurs at about 1,000 milligrams with each meal.

Although it's hard to believe, hot red chilies can also be applied externally to blisters. Numerous studies have shown that the capsaicin squelches herpes blister pain very well. This herb is available in many different ointment preparations, to be dabbed directly on the sore. Be very careful, however, if you try this with cold sores. The ointment is *very hot.* It will bring down the tingly pain very well, but do not allow it to get anywhere else on your face, on any other membrane (if you know what I mean), or in your eye. Apply the ointment with a swab or wash your hands quite thoroughly after dipping your finger. You may want to use detergent, alcohol, or an oil-based product to get absolutely all the oil off your finger.

One more note of caution: While cayenne is an effective antiviral herb, and I rely on it above all others for fast results in herpes outbreaks, traditional systems of holistic healing, including Ayurveda, say that it will actually aggravate inflammation in the long run—read: more blisters. So, in the short run it's good for crisis control, but in the long run it can actually have the opposite effect in susceptible people.

Licorice has a long history of assisting the immune system. This powerful herb can be taken internally or used as an ointment. It is strong anti-inflammatory medicine, with actions comparable to those of cortisone. For herpes blisters, take 3,000 milligrams per day in capsule form. This herb can be a little stool loosening, so work up gradually.

Licorice ointment will contain either the active ingredient glycyrretinic acid or the related compound glycyrrhizic acid. Topical glycyrretinic acid has been shown in clinical studies to reduce pain and healing time. Apply the cream directly to the blister as necessary.

St. John's wort actually has many clinical uses beyond depression. The active ingredient that benefits herpes appears to be hypericin, which researchers now conclude is not the antidepressant component. This herb supports the immune system, reducing viral episodes. Use 3,000 milligrams per day of the whole herb in capsule form or find a preparation standardized for hypericin. The daily dose of a standardized product should contain 1.0 milligram of hypericin per day.

One of the most effective topical treatments for herpes blister outbreaks is simple vitamin E, swabbed directly on the blister. Pierce a vitamin E capsule, squeeze the liquid onto a cotton ball, and place it on the lesion, leaving it in contact as long as possible. Studies have shown that this treatment often brings relief from pain within eight hours, and lesions appear to heal more rapidly.

Many studies have shown that the amino acid lysine is effective at suppressing herpes outbreaks, while the amino acid arginine encourages growth of the virus. Lysine is contained in the body in inverse relationship to arginine. To thwart outbreaks, you need to up your lysine-to-arginine ratio, so add lysine as a supplement and consume lysine-containing foods.

Good lysine foods are beans, brewer's yeast, eggs, milk, potatoes, and most vegetables. At the same time, reduce your consumption of arginine-containing foods, including carob, cereal grains, chocolate, gelatin, nuts, peanuts, raisins, and seeds. Lysine does not cure cold sores, it just prevents outbreaks, so it must be taken in a daily dose to maintain prevention.

To begin lysine supplementation, start with 500 milligrams per day, and work up to the dose that brings total cessation of outbreaks, which is often as high as 3,000 milligrams per day. This dose will frequently minimize the intensity of an outbreak if you begin taking it immediately at the beginning of the prodrome (tingling) phase. Gradually taper down to the amount that will sustain the relief. Often a dose of only 500 milligrams per day will provide total ongoing relief.

Indigestion and Gas

You may not know technically what indigestion is, but I bet you know it when you have it. The term "indigestion," or "upset stomach," refers to a vague collection of gastrointestinal symptoms. "Dyspepsia," the medical label for indigestion, is a catchall term that includes a mixed bag of digestive glitches such as appetite loss, belching, stomach discomfort, gas, bloating, and nausea. Many grave medical conditions can cause tummy suffering, but "dyspepsia" is most often cited when no particular medical cause can be detected. Think of dyspepsia as a stomach version of irritable bowel syndrome, which occurs in the small intestine and colon.

On the whole, clinicians divide indigestion into two categories. The "cold" type is defined by feelings of fullness, slow stomach emptying, and reduced secretions of the digestive organs. This variety feels like "there's a rock in my gut," and often goes along with constipation. Remedies include warming herbs.

The "hot" type of indigestion, or "gastritis," involves inflammation or irritation of the inner lining (mucosa) of the stomach. Gastritis can be caused by many factors and, in some cases, may precede ulcer. Heartburn is a burning sensation caused by stomach acid regurgitating into the esophagus. These people often suffer from diarrhea. Remedies include cooling, soothing herbs.

Traditional herbalists around the world agree that herbs with bitter taste promote digestive secretions and speed up digestion. Gentian root is the most popular "digestive bitter" in Western herbalism. Europeans often drink a "bitter aperitif"—an ounce or so of bitter herbal beverage—before the first bite of a meal, to stimulate digestive secretions and keep food passing through at a good clip. Bitter herbs reduce gas, bloating, symptoms of food allergies, and indigestion. Other bitter digestants include barberry root, dandelion, and artichoke.

For hot, burning, acid indigestion, licorice is good. Licorice guards digestive mucous membranes by increasing production of mucin, a secretion that protects against stomach acid and other digestive juices.[27] In DGL, the glycyrrhizic acid, the ingredient associated with increased blood pressure and water retention, has been removed, but the gastritis-benefiting part of the root has been left intact. One to two chewable wafers of DGL may provide relief.[28]

Peppermint is a well-known herb for tummy troubles. Enteric-coated peppermint oil works well to relieve the symptoms of dyspepsia. Peppermint oil is a relaxant for the muscles of the intestinal wall. Enteric-coating the capsule delays the effect until the remedy is farther down in the digestive tract, as well as reducing peppermint-tasting burps. In one double-blind trial from Taiwan, four out of every five patients experienced reduced symptoms when given enteric-coated peppermint oil.[29] In 1999, a study from Germany used peppermint and caraway oils to test 223 people. The combination brought about a significant reduction in pain.[30] A German study from February 2000 again confirmed that a combination of peppermint and caraway oils effectively reduced the speed of intestinal movement.[31]

Soothing (demulcent) herbs, including marshmallow root (*Althaea officinalis*) and slippery elm bark (*Ulmus fulva*), are high in mucilage, a slimy plant component. Mucilage can be beneficial for people with hot indigestion because its slippery nature soothes an irritated digestive tract. Marshmallow is used for inflammation of the stomach membranes.[32]

For cold, slow, full, alkaline indigestion, carminative herbs are good. These herbs warm up the digestive tract, speed up and increase the thoroughness of digestion, and reduce gas. Fennel, cardamom, dill, cumin and caraway seeds, and lemon balm are carminative.

Tasty, aromatic ginger is a time-tested remedy for stomach upset. It is used by nearly every culture in the world.

Cinnamon bark (*Cinnamomum cassia*) is a warming, mild, but useful remedy for sluggish indigestion. *The Complete German Commission E*

Monographs recommends cinnamon for loss of appetite, dyspeptic complaints, mild gastrointestinal spasm, bloating, and flatulence.

Insomnia

Insomnia is the inability to fall asleep or to stay asleep when appropriate. It's a huge problem for modern Americans. Natural medicine offers many effective short-acting relaxants to help you fall asleep. Let's also look at a few that will help you stay asleep through the night. For the long run, test your pH and begin adjusting your overall body chemistry. You'll be sleeping better in no time.

As its scientific name, *Withania somnifera*, indicates, ashwaganda root aids sleep. Ayurvedic herbalists use the herb to reestablish long-term sleep rhythms. Rather than making you sleepy when you take it, this remedy seems to regulate sleep cycles over time, facilitating more refreshing sleep. Use 1 to 2 grams anytime during the day to restore sleep cycles over time.

Valerian (*Valeriana officinalis*) is a relaxant herb that has a calming effect on the autonomic nervous system. It is a good short-term sedative that works quickly, offering a healthy, nontoxic alternative to strong prescription drugs.[33,34]

For insomnia, valerian is taken right at bedtime to help induce sleep quickly.[35] Valerian is best for insomniacs who have trouble falling asleep because it decreases the amount of time it takes to fall asleep but doesn't necessarily work on the length of sleep.

Because valerian is a mild herb, you may need 3 to 10 grams to get the desired result. Valerian cannot be thought of as a "sleeping pill," which is generally much stronger and requires just one or two tablets. One or two valerian capsules or tablets may work simply to calm nerves, but more may be required as a sleep aid. Start with a lower number and work up till you get the desired result.

Valerian is used widely in Europe, and many of the studies showing its effectiveness were conducted there. In the past thirty-five years, more than 200 scientific studies have been done on valerian. In much of Europe, physicians are more likely to recommend valerian instead of pharmaceuticals. Valerian is an active ingredient in about 150 over-the-counter medicines in Germany, including some preparations for children. (In fact, some studies have shown positive effects on hyperactive children.)

In the United States, it's recommended that valerian not be used by children, pregnant women, or nursing women, except on the advice of a health practitioner.

A typical dose of valerian root, powdered in capsules, is 1,000 to 3,000 milligrams taken several times per day for anxiety and 5,000 milligrams or more taken once a day, before bed, to relax for sleep.

Menstrual Cramps, Premenstrual Syndrome, and Menopause

Female hormone imbalances are common and uncomfortable. Natural medicine has a wealth of cures for these troublesome maladies. Overall, the best long-term strategy is to get your body chemistry balanced and to regain good health. Usually, these female symptoms gradually slip away. We can look at a handful of exceptional remedies for these conditions.

Dong quai root (*Angelica sinensis*), a superb general tonic herb, is the most popular Chinese herb and may be the most extensively used herb in the world, says Christopher Hobbs. Virtually every women in China, as well as millions in other Asian countries, especially Japan, take dong quai daily to strengthen their reproductive organs, regulate their menstrual cycle, and build their health in general. For an energy boost, particularly at vulnerable times of her monthly cycle, an Asian woman might cook an extra bit of dong quai into soup or rice dishes on a daily basis for several days.

Energetically, dong quai is classified as being sweet and pungent. It is mildly warming, with specific strengthening benefits for the heart and liver. Therapeutically, its main function is to build and regulate the blood throughout the body, but especially in the pelvic area, making it particularly valuable in increasing circulation to the female organs. Paul Bergner, clinical director of the Rocky Mountain School of Botanical Studies in Boulder, Colorado, in *The Healing Power of Ginseng* (Prima, 1996), explains that, according to Chinese medicine, pain is often caused by "congealed blood," so the circulation-enhancing qualities of dong quai make it suitable for women's pelvic pain.

Hobbs mentions that dong quai contains coumarins, well-known blood-thinning chemicals, and high levels of vitamin B_{12}, a blood-building nutrient. Other aspects of dong quai chemistry are a bit confusing. While this herb has been used for thousands of years as a female balancing tonic, and many authorities classify it as an estrogenic herb, so far scientific studies have shown no hormonal effect. Clearly, in practical use, however, it works very well to bring balance to hormonal functions. The best theory so far is that it increases circulation to the pelvic organs, notably the ovaries, thus supporting more production of the body's own sex hormones.

For women, dong quai is a medicine cabinet in a jar. Scientific and clinical studies have verified its use in treating premenstrual syndrome (PMS) symptoms including breast tenderness, constipation, and dizziness. It also excels in regulating the period, treating amenorrhea and cramps, and normalizing the blood flow. For menopausal symptoms, women use dong quai when they have hot flashes or pelvic pain.

A study conducted recently by Tori Hudson, N.D., of the National College of Naturopathic Medicine in Portland, Oregon, and Leanna Standish, Ph.D., N.D., of Bastyr University in Seattle, Washington, using dong quai, along with a combination of other herbs, showed a 100 percent result in reducing the severity of menopausal symptoms (hot flashes, insomnia, mood changes, and vaginal dryness).[36]

Dong quai is not just for reproductive organs. Try this herb for high blood pressure, atherosclerosis, asthma, bronchitis, and anemia.

Because it increases blood flow, Bergner recommends dong quai for bruises and the pain of arthritis.

In Chinese herbalism, the typical patient who benefits from dong quai is cold, fatigued, pale, anemic, and in poor overall health. Dong quai comes in many types of preparations, including the famous formula Four Things, in which it is mixed with three additional herbs, including peony. It is available also in a liquid called Tan Kwei Gin that is quite popular. The herb, a member of the parsley family, has a strong celery-like taste and smell, and can be cooked into tasty dishes, such as Dong Quai Soup (see page 173).

Dong quai should not be taken during pregnancy, by overly hot or febrile people, or by those with diarrhea or endometriosis.

Chinese herbal formulas designed to regulate the menstrual cycle or treat PMS almost always center on bupleurum root (*Bupleurum chinense*), a "minor tonic." According to Dan Bensky and Andrew Gamble in *Chinese Herbal Medicine: Materia Medica* (Eastland Press, 1993), the main action of this herb is to relieve blood stagnation in the liver. In women, liver stagnation can cause menstrual cramps, breast swelling, irregular menstrual flow, irritability, and food cravings.

Because bupleurum is relaxing, it can be very helpful in PMS with anxiety and irritability. Its liver-supportive qualities help to reduce sugar cravings, a common PMS symptom.

The energy of bupleurum is bitter and cool, so it's particularly good in women who are always hot or who are developing a fever.

The classic bupleurum patient is a woman who is hot or feverish (maybe with chills), irritable, nauseated, and dizzy, with menstrual pain, high cholesterol, and a tight, sore chest.

White peony root (*Paeonia lactiflora*) is another blood nourisher that supports the liver, which is so important in hormone balance. Bensky and Gamble recommend it to "soften and comfort the liver."

White peony root is a star in the treatment of menopause, for which it is used in Chinese herbalism to treat night sweats, insomnia, and mood swings. Since peony root is a sedative and antispasmodic, it lowers blood pressure, relieves hypertensive headaches, reduces muscle pain, and allows a comfortable night's sleep. Peony is especially known for treating the irregular excessive bleeding of this time of life.

Peony is a very sour, bitter, cool yin and blood tonic. The "peony type" of woman is hot, with muscle cramps in the abdomen, hands, and feet, She has headaches and sweats at night.

White peony root balances well energetically with, and is often used alongside, dong quai and bupleurum.

Pain

We all have pain. Chronic pain, however, is a curse. Generally, excess pain is a sign of the need for detoxification and body balancing. While drugs stop pain fast, they don't solve the problem, and they have side effects. Here are some excellent alternatives.

Corydalis tuber (*yan hu suo*) is nature's medicine for aches and anxiety. It's the main herb used in TCM for treating pain. It is another relative of the poppy, containing isoquinoline alkaloids, mainly tetrahydropalmatine. The raw herb is about 1 percent the strength of opium.[37] Like morphine, it promotes relaxation and relieves pain. While morphine is addictive and creates tolerance, tetrahydropalmatine doesn't have these problems. Chinese herbalists value yan hu suo as a muscle relaxant and use it particularly for menstrual pain.

Several studies in animals have confirmed the benefits of yan hu suo.[38,39] A 1999 animal study performed at the University of Maryland Dental School demonstrated that it significantly reduced pain and inflammation.[40]

Corydalis is relaxing and promotes sleep, so don't take it while driving, and exceed the recommended dose only with caution. Increase the dose gradually until you are familiar with the pain-relieving and sedative effects. As a tea, start with a half ounce of chopped herb, brewed, per day.

Sinus Infection

Ever felt as if someone jammed a boxing glove up your nose? If you've ever had sinusitis, you most certainly have. But it's a pleasure you hope never to repeat. Alas, for many, sinusitis is all too common.

The sinuses are the airspaces within the bones of the face. Sinusitis is an inflammation, due to an infection, within these spaces. If the sinus lining becomes swollen, it can interfere with the normal flow of nasal mucus. Obstructed mucus can fill the sinuses, producing unbearable pressure and an incomparable environment for the growth of invasive bacteria. Allergies can also sow the seeds of infection.

Sinusitis is one of the most common conditions treated by primary-care physicians. An expensive public health issue, it afflicts more than 14 percent of the population—around 35 million Americans—and gobbles up over $2 billion in yearly healthcare costs.

Sinus infection is almost always caused by bacteria. *Streptococcus pneumoniae* is the culprit in about 33 percent of all cases, while *Haemophilus influenzae* generates another quarter of total cases. Acute sinusitis usually accompanies another upper respiratory tract infection such as a cold.

Physicians in this country have long had a practice of prescribing antibiotics to people presenting with infections. The quandary, though, is that most common infections, such as colds, are not caused by bacteria, but by viruses, for which antibiotics are not effective. About 90 percent of sore throats are caused by viral infection, but most are treated with antibiotics. Studies have shown that as many as seven out of ten people are given antibiotics when they seek treatment for common colds. Of patients with sinus symptoms who visit primary-care physicians, one-half to two-thirds are unlikely to have bacterial sinusitis. They probably actually have a cold, for which antibiotics are ineffective. Still, the appropriate function of antibiotics in acute sinusitis treatment is not completely obvious. A recent study of adult patients with acute sinusitis treated with amoxicillin or placebo showed no significant difference in outcomes.

For centuries, herbal medicine has been used in the treatment of common infections. When antibiotic use became widespread in the 1940s, herbal prescribing declined as the "wonder drugs" usurped their place. Botanical medicines function in several powerful ways for sinusitis. Some enhance the body's own natural defenses. Others make it harder for an infection to take hold and stay dug in. Still others have powerful antiviral and antibacterial action.

Since the mid-1800s, *Hydrastis canadensis*, commonly known as goldenseal, has been used throughout the United States. Goldenseal first appeared in mainstream medical literature in 1852 and has maintained a prominent position among leading herbal medicines ever since.

Goldenseal is a premier anti-infection herb. The medicinal value of goldenseal is due to its high content of berberine, which has demonstrated antibacterial and immunostimulatory activity.

Although used for a wide variety of ailments, one of garlic's most significant actions is antimicrobial, due to the potent sulfur compounds it contains. It has been shown to significantly inhibit a number of pathogenic organisms while having little effect on the beneficial intestinal flora. This is an herb whose attributes also support the respiratory system.[41]

An herb seldom used medicinally in the United States, sage (*Salvia officinalis*), has an illustrious history among European herbalists.[42] With its strong antimicrobial action and pleasantly aromatic and mildly pungent taste, sage is often employed as an herbal gargle for adults.

Mainly known as a culinary herb, thyme became popular in the Middle Ages as an antiseptic. Thyme's healing properties stem chiefly from its aromatic oils, thymol and carvacol, which produce strong antibacterial, antifungal, expectorant, and respiratory relaxant activities. The volatile oils direct the main therapeutic benefits to the respiratory system. Thyme is an excellent cough remedy, stimulating the immune system and combating viruses and bacteria simultaneously. Thyme increases the fluidity of phlegm and promotes its expulsion.

Traditional herbal systems value diaphoretics for treating sinus infection. These perspiration-promoting medicines release waste materials and relieve congestion. Peppermint is a classic example. Drink diaphoretics hot.

Cooling diaphoretics are used to reduce fever and inflammation. Chrysanthemum flower and honeysuckle flower (*Lonicera japonica*) are also strongly antimicrobial. Elder flower (*Sambucus nigra*), yarrow flower (*Achillea millefolium*), and boneset leaf (*Eupatorium perfoliatum*) are Western diaphoretics. Noted British herbal authority David Hoffmann calls boneset "the best remedy for the relief of the associated symptoms."[43]

Warming diaphoretics also treat these diseases. Use them when the main symptom is chills. Try basil leaf (*Ocimum spp.*), which is favored in Ayurveda for reducing mucus in the nasal passages.[44,45,46,47] Basil kills bacteria and stimulates the immune system.[48,49] Cinnamon bark is a very effective warming diaphoretic, used at a lower dose, say a half ounce, or in medicinal beverage mixtures.

Another diaphoretic used extensively in Europe but relatively rarely in this country, linden flower (*Tilia cordata*) is used for similar infections. Noted German herbalist Rudolph Weiss reports that an excellent comparative study was done with lime blossom versus antibiotics in childhood respiratory infections. Lime blossom tea was far superior to antibiotics in decreasing the course and severity of the illness.[50]

Urinary Tract Infection

Dr. Lark says that up to 15 percent of women over age sixty have frequent bladder infections. This vicious cycle is well known to precipitate chronic bladder irritation and, eventually, inflammation.

As tissue weakens, it becomes less able to resist infection. Perhaps 25 percent of women have symptom-free bacterial bladder infection. Bacteria use the short female urethra like an entrance chute into the bladder, where they thrive in the warm urine swimming pool. If things deteriorate, these bacteria backstroke their way right into the kidneys, propelling the condition into a life-threatening emergency. A chronic, inflamed infection in the urinary tract is called bacterial cystitis.

Dr. Lee likes the herbal standby cranberry for bladder infection.

Aviva Jill Romm, A.H.G., C.P.M., is a certified professional midwife, practicing registered herbalist, and current president of the American Herbalists Guild. She is the author of several books on natural healing topics, including *Vaccinations: A Thoughtful Parent's Guide* (Inner Traditions, 2001) and *The Natural Pregnancy Book* (Celestial Arts, 2003). Aviva says:

When treating a urinary tract infection, if the typical herbal protocols, including cranberry juice and uva ursi, are not adequate (no significant improvement within 24 hours of commencing treatment), add an oral dose of 2 "00" capsules of baking soda daily along with one of the doses of uva ursi infusion and this will often do the trick. According to the respected German herbalist, Rudolf Fritz Weiss, the alkaline bladder environment created by doing this activates the potential of the uva ursi.

Every normal intestinal tract contains *E. coli* as part of its natural microflora. But these same *E. coli* bacteria can create chaos when they find their way into the wrong place—the urinary tract. More than 80 percent of all bladder infections are caused by *E. coli* entering the urinary tract. This is fifty times more common in women and girls than in men. Dr. Lee uses d-mannose to treat this problem. A simple sugar, d-mannose is closely related to glucose and occurs naturally in cranberry and pineapple juices. Most of it is rapidly absorbed before reaching the intestines, passing through the kidneys and ending up in the urine. Its chemical structure causes it to adhere to the *E. coli*, resulting in bacteria coated by d-mannose in the urine to become unstuck from the bladder wall and be flushed right out of the body. The 1 teaspoon adult dose of d-mannose is substantially more than that in a typical cranberry juice dose. D-mannose is ten times more active than the fructose found in cranberries.

Dr. Lee says, "If the cystitis has a non-infectious etiology, acidic pH in the urine can cause more bladder irritation." She suggests that avoiding acidic foods such as tomatoes, onions, and orange juice can have a beneficial effect. Although these foods are acidic outside the body, they may be influenced by factors other than pH within the body. They may be bladder irritants.

As women age, they often begin consuming less protein, gradually becoming too alkaline. It's important to check pH and adjust before bladder problems, common postmenopausally, become chronic.

Vaginal Infection

The vagina is a perfect breeding ground for infection. Most vaginal infections are caused by pathogenic yeast, but bacteria can also be the villain. The vagina is supposed to be slightly acid (4.0 to 5.0). To treat

Specific Diseases and Treatments / 251

bacteria, adjust the pH of the vagina to be less acidic. For the long term, check pH and adjust your body chemistry overall, as necessary.

To treat yeast, make the vagina more acidic, says Chanchal Cabrera. "I have my patients douche with dilute apple cider vinegar. After the douche, which should only be done occasionally, follow with a capsule or two of acidophilus, inserted as a suppository and left overnight to restore proper flora."[51]

"I do some work balancing vaginal flora with chronic yeast infections by using yogurt as a vaginal wash/suppository," says Aviva Romm. "If the yeast is not clearing up, and if acidophilus suppositories or yogurt washes are not helping or are even aggravating, then acidifying may be the wrong approach."

Boric acid is a mildly antiseptic chemical. A white powder, it is widely available and used for first aid in treating mild microbial (yeast, fungus, some bacteria) infections. Commonly, it is used as a suppository inserted in the vagina to treat yeast infection. Commercial "artificial tears" and eyewash products also may contain boric acid for its antiseptic activity.

In one study, performed at the Department of Obstetrics and Gynecology at New York Hospital, Cornell University Medical Center, 100 women with chronic yeast vaginitis were studied. Their infections had failed to respond to treatment with antifungal medicines, but 98 percent of the women successfully treated their infections with boric acid capsules inserted into the vagina twice per day for two to four weeks.[52]

Another double-blind research paper published in the *American Journal of Obstetrics and Gynecology* reported that 72 percent of the women studied were still cured thirty days after the treatment, while the group treated with nystatin, a common yeast drug, had only a 50 percent rate of cure thirty days later. The women liked the boric acid suppository compared to messy vaginal creams.[53]

Get boric acid powder at the pharmacy. Fill size 00 capsules. The normal dose is two capsules, inserted into the vagina and left overnight. Better to start with a small dose, such as one-third of a capsule, the first time you try this treatment, to make sure all goes well. Side effects are rare, but it's always good to be conservative. Boric acid is toxic. Never ingest it by mouth. To be safe, don't apply it to open wounds. Do not apply it topically to small children.[54]

According to Aviva, lactobacillus overgrowth infections are often mistaken for yeast infections. "Typically most folks will assume yeast, so will treat that first. But lactobacillus infections may not have the typically curdy or yeasty discharge or yeasted bread odor. There may simply be just redness and itching," she says.

If lactobacillus is the culprit, use baking soda capsules to alkalinize the vaginal environment. Try two 00 capules of baking soda inserted nightly into the vaginal vault to see if this clears up the problem.

So how do you know which bug is causing the uproar and which way to push the pH? Just try the antiyeast protocol, and if it doesn't work, switch to the other? Aviva answers, "Well, that is definitely one way to rule out one or the other. Lab analysis is another was to confirm the organism."

Herbs can rival drug treatments in just about every area, even for very difficult conditions. Often, herbal medicines offer options for healing and hope for effective outcomes that conventional methods cannot. Herbal medicine is not a "cute fantasy" or "nice hobby"—it's serious, worthy medicine, and the rest of the world knows it. Unless someone has a genetic disorder, such as Down's syndrome, just about any ailment can be improved with natural medicine. Some, certainly, are more challenging than others, and some will require a variety of interventions.

15

Integrating Herbs and Foods into Daily Life

Now that we've looked at the subject of acid-alkaline balance from all sides, how should you actually proceed with managing your health?

First, be aware. Take a moment every day to assess how you are feeling. Use the principles of Ayurveda, TCM, and the modern understanding of pH to systematically evaluate what's going on in your body and mind. Do you feel energetic? Are you free from pain? Are you sleeping well?

Test It

Initially, you need to test your urine pH daily for many days, to get a consistent average and recognize a pattern. Once you get a sense of how your pH works in your individual body, begin to notice changes from your lifestyle practices. Since you are going to be evaluating your first morning urine, it will have an average of several hours of waste collection. It's a pretty good measure of what you did and ate the day before. Notice any changes from day to day, and think about what happened the day before the change. A weekend sugar binge? A dietary diary (be honest, now) might help.

Now, begin to experiment. Purposely attempt to change your pH. Eat a super acid diet for a couple of days or a week. Any difference? Also be aware of how you feel. Most people will not notice much on this end because their body is working overtime already to pump out maximum buffers and they will just borrow more from the skeleton.

Next, switch to an extremely alkaline program for a similar time. Note the changes. Once you get the hang of what will make a difference in you individually, zero in on a proportion that will keep you in the healthy pH zone.

It takes many months for all these adjustments to fully balance. Make it a habit to honestly assess how you are feeling as the years go by. Filling out a symptom questionnaire every so often—say, once a year—is a great way to put on paper how you are feeling and to remind yourself of any changes. (For a good questionnaire, see the Appendix.) Rating your symptoms will give you some perspective. You may be surprised at how slowly yet extensively your chronic illnesses will improve.

When to Test It

Metabolic wastes accumulate in cycles, according to Asian medicine. You need to assess your health after every meal, every day, every season, and over the course of your life.

The hottest time of the day, on the thermometer and in your cells, is the middle of the day. Your metabolism throws off acids at a high pitch. It's pitta time. That's the time to use cooling alkaline foods and to take a rest, especially if you are a high-acid, hot-tempered type.

Likewise, the hottest season of the year is the summer. Again, this is the season to watch the acid signs. If you begin to feel those telltale signs of acidosis, up your vegetable intake and eat less acid fruit.

Midlife is the hot, intense time for all of us—of course, for some more than others. It's the time when most people who develop inflammatory diseases have their first symptoms. Watch those pitta foods, and emphasize the vata- and kapha-promoting diets.

How to Live It

Making all these changes isn't always easy. For some, they are pretty radical. Giving up white sugar is usually very difficult. People get used to it as a source of quick energy. It's always available. Everyone else is gobbling it down. It's tasty and legal.

These changes need to be gradual. When I see someone make a decision to become a natural health fanatic and go home, clean out all the cupboards, and dump all the "bad" foods in the garbage, I see someone whose cupboards will soon be filled right back up with the very same products. This person doesn't know what to eat instead of those discarded foods. How do you prepare aduki beans, anyway?

Start with one change that you can manage. If it's gradually reducing white sugar over a couple of months until you're not using it at all, great. If it's transitioning to cooking with whole grains over three months while you get the hang of the new ingredients, that's progress.

It's all about getting in the habit of thinking this way and letting that mind-set become your lifestyle. Natural foods cooking requires a bit of extra planning, but not necessarily a lot of extra time. Start thinking about your new regime before you go to the store. Make a list. Stick to it. Add a few new items each time and gradually switch over.

You need to plan. The moment you arrive home late, after a grueling day at the office, is not the time to start the soybeans boiling on the stove. Instead, fill your refrigerator in advance with healthy foods that you know will balance your pH needs. Select foods that are reasonable to prepare with your schedule. Prepare larger quantities in advance and use them up over a few meals. Do some prep work on the weekend. (That's the time to have the dried beans boiling—while you're cleaning the garage on Saturday afternoon.)

Since the main thrust of pH eating for most people is to drastically up the vegetable content, start with vegetables that you can cook quickly and simply. The first time you try preparing fresh beets and find yourself peeling them for an hour and then cleaning up red juice from all over your kitchen, you will reach for the microwave burgers. Zucchini is a simple vegetable that cooks quickly and tastes good. When you get home, already exhausted, you can simply slice them and put them on the stove to steam. Go hit the shower. By the time you return to the kitchen, dinner will be ready. Add some soy sauce and a little crushed dill, and enjoy.

Celery is one of the most alkalinizing vegetables you can eat. It's definitely underappreciated in the United States. Considered the most cooling and anti-inflammatory food we have, it is an excellent nerve nutrient. It is so relaxing that a glass of celery juice can put you to sleep. Celery juice was our standby for drug-withdrawal insomnia at the hospital. At home, you can steam celery as a side dish. Again, it's extremely simple to prepare. Chop, steam, done. Add sauce. Savor. Mix the steamed celery with other vegetables for a flavor medley if you prefer. Or add it raw to salads.

Drink herbal teas every day. Most tea herbs are alkalinizing. Consult an herb book by an authoritative author (see the Recommended Reading list on page 279 for suggestions). Select one or more mild medicinal teas that match your long-term health needs or a variety of herbal beverage teas that appeal to you. Brew a strong pot in the morning and savor several cups during the day. Take herb tea to work with you as a substitute for soft drinks.

Drink Yogi Tea (see page 175) regularly. This special Ayurvedic blend is used by yoga practitioners to maintain stamina and good digestion, and support the immune system. In my house, we make this tea in large batches and drink it every day. It's also available in teabags in health food stores and grocery stores.

Exercise every day. Movement helps the muscles and other tissues shed their acid burden. Increasing your breathing dumps carbon dioxide. Check out your Ayurvedic constitution and adapt your program to complement your body's ideal exercise needs.

Acid-alkaline balance is the most overlooked health-enhancing factor in modern medicine, conventional or alternative. It has been methodically disregarded by modern practitioners for a century. Even though it has an obvious correlation with the health of all of us, the study of pH has never evolved into a major focus of attention.

We all depend on proper pH for life. The clinical use, and the personal home use, of pH techniques gives all of us a very important key to be optimally healthy in body, mind, and mood. Now that you understand pH concepts, you know how to bring yourself into balance. You have the tools to avoid disease. You're in on the secret knowledge that is so critical for proper health. Understanding pH can, and will, keep you well.

Now you know how Dr. X and Dr. Y can both be right. But are they right for you? Figure it out for yourself. Individualization is the key. We all have different bodies, each with different strengths and weaknesses, so we all need different strategies to get well and stay well.

With the knowledge you have now gained, you can achieve balanced health. And a balanced body can be more powerful than disease for the long run. After all, natural healing is all about prevention. The study of acid-alkaline balance is the ultimate preventive self-care health system.

The techniques of self-care of the Body Balance program are aimed at never allowing you to have a symptom and, if you do, to bringing you back into balance quickly and effectively, so that you don't have another.

You're not far from that time when you're free from sickness, when you haven't been troubled by even a sore throat or headache for years. That future will soon become your reality. I've personally watched hundreds of folks build energetic health and stamina. Body Balance is a different vision of the vibrant human—not just the slowly ailing, wailing, failing human, but an energetic, exciting being with energy to excel. By learning and applying the methods in this book, you will manifest that type of radiant good health.

In my long hunt for a coherent, consistent theory that explains the success of the bewildering plethora of health programs, I became convinced that acid-alkaline balance was a big part of the answer. I think you will find the same.

Through pH techniques, we have been given a measuring tool that average people can master and apply. Acid-alkaline balance answers all those pesky questions like, "Why do some people do better on a low-fat diet, while others can tolerate fat by the bucket?" Body Balance is the glue that holds all the various speculations, traditions, and techniques together. As you begin to take steps to live the life that only you can live—nourishing your body with an individualized, tailored diet, based on Body Balance principles, and building on that foundation with herbs, foods, and teas to heal illness, soothe injury, and tip the odds against disease and degeneration in your favor—you will enter a whole new world of excellence and high spirits, with energy you never knew you could have. My most heartfelt best wishes to you as you create a world where your life is abundant, your mind is blissful, and your body is beautiful.

APPENDIX: PERSONAL BODY BALANCE QUESTIONNAIRE

I. Acid Producers

	Rarely (1 point)	Occasionally (2 points)	Often (3 points)
Do you eat red meat more than twice a week?			
Do you consume more than one serving of milk product daily?			
Do you eat fried foods?			
Do you eat white sugar?			
Do you drink caffeinated beverages?			
Do you drink alcohol?			
Do you have food allergies?			
Do you experience daily emotional stress?			
Do you exert yourself physically to the point of exhaustion or pain?			
Do you use over-the-counter remedies for upset stomach?			
Are you fatigued, even after enough hours of sleep?			
Are you in or past midlife?			
Do you have joint pain?			

I. Acid Producers (Continued)			
	Rarely (1 point)	Occasionally (2 points)	Often (3 points)
Do you have frequent heartburn?			
Do you have frequent colds and flu?			
Do you have acne, irritability, dizziness, depression, memory loss, or insomnia?			
Do you have "hot" asthma?			
Do you have chronic inflammation (bursitis, tendonitis, colitis)?			
Do you have chronic urinary tract infection?			
Do you have low libido, PMS, diarrhea, mal-odorous urine, headache, or rapid breathing?			
Total points in each column			

Total the points from all three columns. The higher your score, the more you are in danger of acidosis. Check your pH.

II. Alkaline Producers

	Rarely (1 point)	Occasionally (2 points)	Often (3 points)
Do you eat at least five servings of fruits and vegetables daily?			
Do you limit your grains to whole forms (whole wheat, etc.)?			
Do you drink plenty of water?			
Do you have chronic low body temperature?			
Do you chronically have excessive, cold, thick, opaque, or goopy mucus?			
Do you have "wet" asthma?			
Do you take a break to relax and enjoy your life at least once a day?			
Do you meditate?			
Do you get plenty of sleep, and awaken refreshed?			
Do you have bone spurs or plantar fasciitis?			
Do you have edema (especially in your hands)?			
Do you have numbness or prickling sensations?			
Do you have "full"-type indigestion (decreased stomach acid)?			
Total points in each column			

Total the points from all three columns. The higher your score, the more you are in danger of alkalosis. Check your pH.

III. Do You Need a Detox?

	Rarely (1 point)	Occasionally (2 points)	Often (3 points)
Are you fatigued or lethargic?			
Do you have concentration problems or fuzzy thinking?			
Do you experience depression?			
Do you have mood swings?			
Do you have frequent colds?			
Do you have congestion or a stuffy nose?			
Do you have bad breath?			
Do you have a coated tongue?			
Do you have a bitter or metallic taste in your mouth?			
Do you have a strong or offensive body odor?			
Do you have strong-smelling urine?			
Do you experience insomnia?			
Do you feel unrefreshed upon waking?			
Do you have body aches and pains?			

III. DO YOU NEED A DETOX? (Continued)			
	Rarely (1 point)	Occasionally (2 points)	Often (3 points)
Do you have weak or brittle nails?			
Do you have dark circles under your eyes?			
Do you experience bloating or gas?			
Do you experience indigestion?			
Do you have less than one bowel movement per day?			
Do you have chronic anxiety?			
Do you have food or chemical sensitivity?			
Do you have allergies?			
Do you have eczema or skin rashes?			
Are you overweight?			
Does dietary fiber cause constipation?			
Total points in each column			

Total the points from all three columns. The higher your score, the more your need for a thorough detoxification program. Check your pH, see your healthcare practitioner, and begin to clean out. Remember, most "toxins" are acids, so you might need to follow an alkalinizing program.

NOTES

Chapter 1
1. Personal communication.
2. Personal communication.
3. http://www.drlark.com.
4. http://www.drlark.com.

Chapter 4
1. Naboru Muramoto, *Healing Ourselves* (New York: Avon, 1973).

Chapter 5
1. Personal communication.

Chapter 7
1. "Acid, Base and pH Tutorial," *Technology Studies in Education Research Portal*, http://lrs.ed.uiuc.edu/students/erlinger/water/background/ph.html.
2. *pH of Common Substances*, http://crystal.biol.csufresno.edu:8080/~davidz/Chem3AF97/ChP/CommonpH.html.
3. "pH Table," *Miami Museum of Science*, http://www.miamisci.org/ph/hhoh.html.

Chapter 8
1. Amanda Onion, "Glucose + Oxygen = Smarts," *ABC News.com*, April 2, 2001, http://abcnews.go.com/sections/living/DailyNews/bloodoxygen010402.html.
2. R. Wiley, "The Effect of Acid-Alkaline Nutrition on Psychophysiological

Function," *International Journal of Biosocial Research*, vol. 9, no. 2 (1987): 182–202.

3. S. J. Schoenthaler, "The Northern California Diet-Behaviour Program: An Empirical Evaluation of 3000 Incarcerated Juveniles in Stanislaus County Juvenile Hall," *International Journal of Biosocial Research*, vol. 5, no. 2 (1983): 99–106.

4. Theodore A. Baroody, *Alkalize or Die* (Waynesville, NC: Holographic Health, 1991), p. 22.

5. K. D. Cashman, "Calcium Intake, Calcium Bioavailability and Bone Health," *British Journal of Nutrition*, vol. 87, Suppl. 2 (2002): S169–77.

6. Personal communication.

7. William Lee Cowden, "The Harmful Effects of an Imbalanced pH on the Body Systems," *Nature's Sunshine Products National Convention*, 2003.

8. Personal communication.

9. Personal communication.

10. *Health Equations*, http://healthequations.com/products.html.

11. D. A. Bushinsky, "Acid-Base Imbalance and the Skeleton," *European Journal of Nutrition*, vol. 40, no. 5 (Oct. 2001): 238–44.

12. S. J. Whiting and H. H. Draper, "Effect of a Chronic Acid Load as Sulfate or Sulfur Amino Acids on Bone Metabolism in Adult Rats," *Journal of Nutrition*, vol. 111, no. 10 (1981): 1721–26.

13. K. L. Tucker, H. Chen, M. T. Hannan, L. A. Cupples, P. W. Wilson, D. Felson, and D. P. Kiel, "Bone Mineral Density and Dietary Patterns in Older Adults: The Framingham Osteoporosis Study," *American Journal of Clinical Nutrition*, vol. 76, no. 1 (2002): 245–52.

14. S. Liu, J. E. Manson, I. M. Lee, S. R. Cole, C. H. Hennekens, W. C. Willett, and J. E. Buring, "Fruit and Vegetable Intake and Risk of Cardiovascular Disease: The Women's Health Study," *American Journal of Clinical Nutrition*, vol. 72, no. 4 (2000): 922–28.

15. V. Mijatovic and M. J. van der Mooren, "Homocysteine in Postmenopausal Women and the Importance of Hormone Replacement Therapy," *Clinical Chemistry and Laboratory Medicine*, vol. 39, no. 8 (2001): 764–67.

16. C. L. Krumdieck and C. W. Prince, "Mechanisms of Homocysteine Toxicity on Connective Tissues: Implications for the Morbidity of Aging," *Journal of Nutrition*, vol. 130, no. 2S, Suppl (2000): 365S–68S.

17. Lee Scheier, "Salicylic Acid: One More Reason to Eat Your Fruits and Vegetables," *Journal of the American Dietetic Association*, http://www.find articles.com/cf_0/m0822/12_101/80949235/p1/article. jhtml, Dec, 2001.

18. L. A. Frassetto, E. Nash, R. C. Morris Jr, and A. Sebastian, "Comparative

Effects of Potassium Chloride and Bicarbonate on Thiazide-Induced Reduction in Urinary Calcium Excretion," *Kidney International*, vol. 58, no. 2 (2000): 748–52.

19. Personal communication.

20. Altha Roberts Edgren, "Respiratory Acidosis," *Gale Encyclopedia of Medicine*, http://www.findarticles.com/cf_0/g2601/0011/2601001178/p1/article. jhtml?term=pH+balance.

21. Personal communication.

22. "Fecal Analysis in the Diagnosis of Intestinal Dysbiosis," *The Regence Insurance Group*, http://www.nwmb.org/trgmedpol/laboratory/lab35.html.

Chapter 9

1. http://www.ostex.com/.

2. I. Gorai, Y. Taguchi, O. Chaki, M. Nakayama, and H. Minaguchi, "Specific Changes of Urinary Excretion of Cross-Linked N-Telopeptides of Type I Collagen in Pre- and Postmenopausal Women: Correlation with Other Markers of Bone Turnover," *Calcified Tissue International*, vol. 60 (1997): 317–22.

3. Michael Schachter, "Introduction to the Digestive System," *Health World*, http://www.healthy.net/asp/templates/article.asp?PageType=Article&ID=538.

4. "About the Gastrogram Study," *Asheville Integrative Medicine*, http://www.integrative-med.com/TOPICS/subtopics/gastrogram.html.

5. "Resting for Stomach Acidity," *Total Wellness*, http://www.healthfacts.net/demo/ diet/Acid_Test-F.htm.

6. http://www.nutri-spec.net/started.htm.

7. "Comprehensive Digestive Stool Analysis," http://www.gsdl.com/assessments/cdsa/appguide.

Chapter 10

1. A. Sebastian, L. A. Frassetto, D. E. Sellmeyer, R. L. Merriam, and R. C. Morris Jr., "Estimation of the Net Acid Load of the Diet of Ancestral Preagricultural Homo Sapiens and Their Hominid Ancestors," *American Journal of Clinical Nutrition*, vol. 76, no. 6 (Dec. 2002): 1308–16.

2. Michael A. Schmidt, *Smart Fats* (Berkeley, CA: North Atlantic Books, 1997).

3. Robert Young and Shelley Young, *The pH Miracle* (New York: Warner, 2002).

4. P. B. Rapuri, J. C. Gallagher, H. K. Kinyamu, and K. L. Ryschon, "Caffeine Intake Increases the Rate of Bone Loss in Elderly Women and

Interacts with Vitamin D Receptor Genotypes," *American Journal of Clinical Nutrition,* vol. 74, no. 5 (2001): 694–700.

5. *Health Equations,* http://healthequations.com/articles.htm.

6. M. K. Li, J. P. Kavanagh, V. Prendiville, A. Buxton, D. G. Moss, and N. J. Blacklock, "Does Sucrose Damage Kidneys?" *British Journal of Urology,* vol. 58, no. 4 (1986): 353–57.

7. M. G. Holl and L. H. Allen, "Sucrose Ingestion, Insulin Response and Mineral Metabolism in Humans," *Journal of Nutrition,* vol. 117, no. 7 (1987): 1229–33.

8. N. U. Nguyen, M. T. Henriet, G. Dumoulin, A. Widmer, and J. Regnard, "Increase in Calciuria and Oxaluria After a Single Chocolate Bar Load," *Hormone and Metabolic Research,* vol. 26, no. 8 (1994): 383–86.

9. M. G. Holl and L. H. Allen, "Sucrose Ingestion, Insulin Response and Mineral Metabolism in Humans," *Journal of Nutrition,* vol. 117, no. 7 (1987): 1229–33.

10. K. L. Tucker, H. Chen, M. T. Hannan, L. A. Cupples, P. W. Wilson, D. Felson, and D. P. Kiel, "Bone Mineral Density and Dietary Patterns in Older Adults: The Framingham Osteoporosis Study," *American Journal of Clinical Nutrition,* vol. 76, no.1 (2002): 245–52.

11. J. Salmeron, J. E. Manson, M. J. Stampher, G. A. Colditz, A. L. Wing, and W. C. Willett, "Dietary Fiber, Glycemic Load, and Risk of Non-Insulin-Dependent Diabetes Mellitus in Women." *Journal of the American Medical Association,* vol. 277, no. 6 (Feb. 12, 1977): 472–77.

12. L. S. Augustin, L. Dal Maso, C. La Vecchia, M. Parpinel, E. Negri, S. Vaccarella, C. W. Kendall, D. J. Jenkins, and S. Francesch, "Dietary Glycemic Index and Glycemic Load, and Breast Cancer Risk: A Case-Control Study," *Annals of Oncology,* vol. 12, no. 11 (Nov. 2001): 1533–38.

13. "Whole Grain Food Intake May Reduce Risk of Diabetes and Cardiovascular Disease," *Integrative Medicine,* http://www.onemedicine.com/News/NewsBrief/DisplayNewsBriefs.asp?Main=newsandarticles&Item=news#1.

14. N. M. McKeown, J. B. Meigs, S. Liu, P. W. Wilson, and P. F. Jacques, "Whole-Grain Intake Is Favorably Associated with Metabolic Risk Factors for Type 2 Diabetes and Cardiovascular Disease in the Framingham Offspring Study," *American Journal of Clinical Nutrition,* vol. 76, no. 2 (2002): 390–98.

15. S. Franceschi, A. Favero et al., "Intake of Macronutrients and Risk of Breast Cancer," *Lancet,* vol. 18, no. 5 (1996): 1351-56.

16. What Is Salt?" *Salt Institute,* http://www.saltinstitute.org/15.html.

17. Jeanne Rattenbury, "The Sea Salt Scene," *Vegetarian Times,* April 1995, http://www.findarticles.com/cf_dls/m0820/n212/16845832/print.jhtml.

18. The Grain and Salt Society, http://www.celtic-seasalt.com/index.html.

19. http://healthequations.com/articles.html#.

20. J. P. Midgley, A. G. Matthew, C. M. Greenwood, and A. G. Logan, "Effect of Reduced Dietary Sodium on Blood Pressure: A Meta-Analysis of Randomized Controlled Trials," *Journal of the American Medical Association*, vol. 27, no. 20 (1996): 1590–97.

21. Wyshak, G., "Teenaged Girls, Carbonated Beverage Consumption, and Bone Fractures," *Archives of Pediatrics and Adolescent Medicine*, vol. 154, no. 6 (June 2000): 610–13.

22. F. Garcia-Contreras, R. Paniagua, M. Avila-Diaz, L. Cabrera-Munoz, I. Martinez-Muniz, E. Foyo-Niembro, and D. Amato. "Cola Beverage Consumption Induces Bone Mineralization Reduction in Ovariectomized Rats," *Archives of Medical Research*, vol. 31, no. 4 (Jul-Aug 2000): 360–65.

23. L. Frassetto, R. C. Morris Jr., D. E. Sellmeyer, K. Todd, and A. Sebastian, "Diet, Evolution and Aging—The Pathophysiologic Effects of the Post-Agricultural Inversion of the Potassium-to-Sodium and Base-to-Chloride Ratios in the Human Diet," *European Journal of Nutrition*, vol. 40 (2001): 200–13.

24. Bernard Jensen, *Nature Has a Remedy* (Escondido, CA: Bernard Jensen Publications, 1978), p. 18.

Chapter 11

1. D. A. Drossman, Z. Li et al, "U.S. Householder Survey of Functional Gastrointestinal Disorders: Prevalence, Sociodemography, and Health Impact," *Digestive Diseases and Sciences*, vol. 38, no. 9 (1993): 1569–80.

2. R. H. Dowling, M. J. Veysey, S. P. Pereira, S. H. Hussaini, L. A. Thomas, J.A.H. Wass, and G. M. Murphy, "Role of Intestinal Transit in the Pathogenesis of Gallbladder Stones," *Canadian Journal of Gastroenterology*, vol. 11 no. 1 (1997): 57–64.

3. Michael T. Murray, *Natural Alternatives to Over-the-Counter and Prescription Drugs* (New York: William Morrow and Company, 1994), p. 56.

4. T. Mitsuoka, H. Hidaka, and T. Eida, "Effect of Fructo-Oligosaccharides on Intestinal Microflora," *Nahrung*, vol. 31, no. 5–6 (1987): 427–36.

5. J. H. Cummings, S. Christie, and T. J. Cole, "A Study of Fructo Oligosaccharides in the Prevention of Travellers' Diarrhea," *Alimentary Pharmacology and Therapeutics*, vol. 15, no. 8 (2001): 1139–45.

6. Y. Bouhnik, B. Flourie, M. Riottot, N. Bisetti, M. F. Gailing, A. Guibert, F. Bornet, and J. C. Rambaud, "Effects of Fructo-Oligosaccharides Ingestion on Fecal Bifidobacteria and Selected Metabolic Indexes of Colon Carcinogenesis in Healthy Humans," *Nutrition and Cancer*, vol. 26, no. 1 (1996): 21–29.

7. I. Chakurski, M. Matev, A. Koichev, I. Angelova, and G. Stefanov,

"Treatment of Chronic Colitis with an Herbal Combination of Taraxacum Officinale, Hipericum Perforatum, Melissa Officinaliss, Calendula Officinalis and Foeniculum Vulgare," *Vutreshni Bolesti*, vol. 20, no. 6 (1981): 51–54.

8. Michael T. Murray, *The Healing Power of Herbs* (Rocklin, CA: Prima, 1995).

9. Michael T. Murray and Joseph Pizzorno, *Encyclopedia of Natural Medicine* (Rocklin, CA: Prima, 1998).

10. R. Patacchini, C. A. Maggi, and A. Meli, "Capsaicin-like Activity of Some Natural Pungent Substances on Peripheral Endings of Visceral Primary Afferents," *Naunyn-Schmiedebergs-Arch-Pharmacol*, vol. 342, no. 1 (1990): 72–77.

11. A. Rasyid and A. Lelo, "The Effect of Curcumin and Placebo on Human Gall-Bladder Function: An Ultrasound Study," *Alimentary Pharmacology and Therapeutics*. vol. 13 (1999): 245–49.

12. H. P. Ammon and M. A. Wahl, "Pharmacology of Curcuma Longa," *Planta Medica*, vol. 57 (1991): 1–7.

13. V. Thamlikitkul, N. Bunyapraphatsara, et al., "Randomized Double Blind Study of *Curcuma Domestica Val.* for Dyspepsia," *Journal of the Medical Association of Thailand*, vol. 72 (1989): 613–20.

14. "WHO Monographs on Selected Medicinal Plants," *World Health Organization*, Geneva, 1999.

15. Y. Goso, Y. Ogata, K. Ishihara, and K Hotta, "Effects of Traditional Herbal Medicine on Gastric Acid," *Biochemi und Physiologie der Pflanzen*, vol. 113C (1996): 17–21.

16. P. I. Reed and W. A. Davies, "Controlled Trial of a Carbenoxolone/Alginate Antacid Combination in Reflux Oesophagitis," *Current Medical Research and Opinion*, vol. 5 (1978) : 637–44.

17. J. H. Liu, G. H. Chen, H. Z. Yeh, C. K Huang, and S. K. Poon, "Enteric-Coated Peppermint-Oil Capsules in the Treatment of Irritable Bowel Syndrome: A Prospective, Randomized Trial," *Journal of Gastroenterology*, vol. 32, no. 6 (1997): 765–68.

18. J. Freise and S. Kohler, "Peppermint Oil-Caraway Oil Fixed Combination in Non-Ulcer Dyspepsia—Comparison of the Effects of Enteric Preparations," *Pharmazie*, vol. 54, no. 3 (1999): 210–15.

19. G. H. Micklefield, I. Greving, and B. May, "Effects of Peppermint Oil and Caraway Oil on Gastroduodenal Motility," *Phytotherapy Research*, vol. 14, no. 1 (2000): 20–23.

20. Robert S. McCaleb, *Herb Research Foundation Encyclopedia of Popular Herbs* (Roseville, CA: Prima, 2000).

21. G. H. Micklefield, I. Greving, and B. May, op. cit.

22. Ibid.

Chapter 12

1. D. M. Eisenberg, R. C. Kessler, C. Foster, F. E. Norlock, D. R. Calkins, and T. L. Delbanco, "Unconventional Medicine in the United States: Prevalence, Costs, and Patterns of Use," *New England Journal of Medicine*, vol. 382 (1993): 246–52.

2. J. Borkan, J. O. Neher, O. Anson, and B. Smoker, "Referrals for Alternative Therapies," *Journal of Family Practice*, vol. 39 (1994): 545–50.

3. J. A. Astin, "Why Patients Use Alternative Medicine," *Journal of the American Medical Association*, vol. 279 (1998): 1548–53.

4. Personal communication.

Chapter 13

1. James A. Duke, *The Green Pharmacy* (Emmaus, PA: Rodale, 1997).

2. A. S. Abdul Ghani and R. Amin, "The Vascular Action of Aqueous Extracts of Foeniculum Vulgare Leaves," *Journal of Ethnopharmacology*, vol. 24, no. 2–3 (1988): 213–18.

3. Paul Pitchford, *Healing with Whole Foods* (Berkeley, CA: North Atlantic Books, 1993).

4. M. Blumenthal, et al., eds., *The Complete German Commission E Monographs.* (Austin, TX: Integrative Medicine Communications, 1998).

5. Cass Ingram, *Supermarket Remedies* (Buffalo Grove, IL: Knowledge House, 1998).

6. K. J. Lachowicz, G. P. Jones, D. R. Briggs, F. E. Bienvenu, J. Wan, A. Wilcock, and M. J. Coventry, "The Synergistic Preservative Effects of the Essential Oils of Sweet Basil (*Ocimum Basilicum L.*) Against Acid-Tolerant Food Microflora," *Letters in Applied Microbiology*, vol. 26, no. 3 (1998): 209–14.

7. K. Karthikeyan, P. Ravichandran, and S. Govindasamy, "Chemopreventive Effect of Ocimum Sanctum on DMBA-Induced Hamster Buccal Pouch Carcinogenesis," *Oral Oncology*, vol. 35, no. 1 (1999): 112–19.

8. A. Singh and A. R. Rao, "Evaluation of the Modulatory Influence of Black Pepper (*Piper nigrum, L.*) on the Hepatic Detoxication System," *Cancer Letters*, vol. 72, no. 1–2 (1993): 5–9.

9. I. Kaoul and A. Kapil. "Evaluation of the Liver Protective Potential of Piperine, an Active Principal of Black and Long Peppers," *Planta Medica*, vol. 59 (1993): 413–17.

10. A. Khajuria, U. Zutshi, and K. L. Bedi, "Permeability Characteristics of Piperine on Oral Absorption—An Active Alkaloid from Peppers and a Bioavailability Enhancer," *Indian Journal of Experimental Biology*, vol. 36, no. 1 (1998): 46–50.

11. G. Shoba, D Joy, T. Joseph, M. Majeed, R Rajendran, and P.S. Srinivas,

"Influence of Piperine on the Pharmacokinetics of Curcumin in Animals and Human Volunteers," *Planta Medica*, vol. 64, no. 4 (1998): 353–56.

12. K. R. Shanmugasundaram, et al., "Amritabindu for Depletion of Antioxidants," *Journal of Ethnopharmacology*, vol. 42, no. 2 (1994): 83–93.

13. Yogi Bhajan, *The Ancient Art of Self-Healing* (Eugene, OR: Silver Streak Publishers, 1982).

14. A. Bordia, et al., "Effect of Ginger (*Zingiber Officinale Rose*) and Fenugreek (*Trigonella Foenumgraecum L.*) on Blood Lipids, Blood Sugar and Platelet Aggregation in Patients with Coronary Artery Disease," *Prostaglandins, Leukotrienes and Essential Fatty Acids*, vol. 58, no. 5 (1997): 379–84.

15. David Hoffmann, *The New Holistic Herbal* (Longmead, England: Element, 1983).

16. P. Mittman, "Randomized, Double-Blind Study of Freeze-Dried Urtica Dioica in the Treatment of Allergic Rhinitis," *Planta Medica*, vol. 56, no. 1 (1990): 44–47.

17. John Heinerman, *Encyclopedia of Fruits, Vegetables, and Herbs* (New York: Parker, 1988).

18. S. Chrubasik, E. Eisenberg, E. Balan, T. Weinberger, R. Luzzati, and C. Conradt, "Treatment of Low Back Pain Exacerbations with Willow Bark Extract: A Randomized Double-Blind Study," *American Journal of Medicine*, vol. 109, no. 1 (2000): 9–14.

19. M. Blumenthal, et al., eds., *The Complete German Commission E Monographs*. (Austin, TX: Integrative Medicine Communications, 1998).

20. G. Nosal'ova, A. Strapkova, A. Kardosova, P. Capek, L. Zathurecky, and E. Bukovska, "Antitussive Action of Extracts and Polysaccharides of Marsh Mallow (*Althea Officinalis L.*, Var. *Robusta*)," *Pharmazie*, vol. 47, no. 3 (1992): 224–26.

21. J. Serkedjieva, "Combined Antiinfluenza Virus Activity of Flos Verbasci Infusion and Amantadine Derivatives," *Phytotherapy Research*, vol. 14, no. 7 (2000): 571–74.

22. I. Zgorniak-Nowosielska, J. Grzybek, N. Manolova, J. Serkedjieva, and B. Zawilinska, "Antiviral Activity of Flos Verbasci Infusion Against Influenza and Herpes Simplex Viruses," *Archivum Immunologiae et Therapiae Experimentalis (Warsz)*, vol. 39, no. 1–2 (1991): 103–8.

23. E. M. Sarrell, A. Mandelberg, and H. A. Cohen, "Efficacy of Naturopathic Extracts in the Management of Ear Pain Associated with Acute Otitis Media," *Archives of Pediatric and Adolescent Medicine*, vol. 155, no. 7 (2001): 796–99.

24. "Willow Bark Monograph," European Scientific Cooperative on Phytotherapy Monographs, Exeter, UK, 1997.

25. "Willow Bark Monograph," American Herbal Pharmacopoeia, Santa Cruz, CA, 1999.

26. Robert S. McCaleb, *Herb Research Foundation Encyclopedia of Popular Herbs* (Roseville, CA: Prima, 2000).

27. Simon Mills and Kerry Bone, *Principles and Practice of Phytotherapy* (London: Churchill Livingstone, 2000).

28. M. Blumenthal, W. R Busse, et al., eds., op. cit.

Chapter 14

1. *Acta Diabetologica*, vol. 52 (1972): 141–45.

2. *PDR for Herbal Medicines* (Montvale, NJ: Medical Economics Company, 1998).

3. A. Rolland, J. Fleurentin, M. C. Lanhers, C. Younos, R. Misslin, F. Mortier, and J. M. Pelt, "Behavioural Effects of the American Traditional Plant Eschscholzia Californica: Sedative and Anxiolytic Properties," *Planta Medica*, vol. 57, no. 3 (1991): 212–16.

4. J. M. Herbert, J. M. Augereau, J. Gleye, and J. P. Maffrand, "Chelery-thrine Is a Potent and Specific Inhibitor of Protein Kinase C," *Biochemical and Biophysical Research Communications*, vol. 172, no. 3 (1990): 993–99.

5. S. T. Meller, C. Dykstra, and G. F. Gebhart, "Acute Thermal Hyper-algesia in the Rat Is Produced by Activation of N-Methyl-D-Aspartate Receptors and Protein Kinase C and Production of Nitric Oxide," *Neuroscience*, vol. 71. no. 2 (1996): 327–35.

6. C. Reimeier, I. Schneider, W. Schneider, H. L. Schafer. and E. F. Elstner, "Effects of Ethanolic Extracts from Eschscholtzia Californica and Corydalis Cava on Dimerization and Oxidation of Enkephalins," *Arzneimittel-forschung*, vol. 45, no. 2 (1995): 132–36.

7. *National Institute of Ayurvedic Medicine*, New York, http://www.niam.com.

8. Jonathan V. Wright, "Fifty Years of Canker Sore Misery and the Simple Treatment That Ended Them," *Health News and Review*, vol. 4, no. 3 (1994): 2.

9. Y. Ozaki, "Antiinflammatory Effect of Tetramethylpyrazine and Ferulic Acid," *Chemical and Pharmaceutical Bulletin*, vol. 40, no. 4 (1992): 954–56.

10. C. R. Shao, F. M. Chen, and Y. X. Tang, "Clinical and Experimental Study on Ligusticum Wallichii Mixture in Preventing and Treating Bronchial Asthma," *Zhongguo Zhong Xi Yi Jie He Za Zhi*, vol. 14, no. 8 (1994): 465–68.

11. D. Bensky and A. Gamble, *Chinese Herbal Medicine: Materia Medica* (Seattle, WA: Eastland Press; 1986), pp. 383–84.

12. James A. Duke, *The Green Pharmacy* (Emmaus, PA: Rodale, 1997).

13. J. Hotz and K. Plein, "Effectiveness of Plantago Seed Husks in Comparison with Wheat Brain on Stool Frequency and Manifestations of Irritable

Colon Syndrome with Constipation," *Medizinische Klinik*, vol. 89, no. 12 (1994): 645–51.

14. A. Prior and P. J. Whorwell, "Double Blind Study of Ispaghula in Irritable Bowel Syndrome," *Gut*, vol. 28, no. 11 (1987): 1510–13.

15. A. Kumar, N. Kumar, J. C. Vij, S. K. Sarin, and B. S. Anand, "Optimum Dosage of Ispaghula Husk in Patients with Irritable Bowel Syndrome: Correlation of Symptom Relief with Whole Gut Transit Time and Stool Weight," *Gut*, vol. 28, no. 2 (1987): 150–55.

16. M. Blumenthal, et al., eds., *The Complete German Commission E Monographs*. (Austin, TX: Integrative Medicine Communications, 1998), p. 167.

17. *Pharmazie*, vol 13 (1958): 423–35.

18. *Wiener Medizinische Wocheschrift*, vol. 1223 (1975): 705–9.

19. *Herbal Medications* (Priest and Priest, Fowler and Co., 1982).

20. *Journal of Pharmacy and Pharmacology*, vol. 25 (1973): 447–52.

21. *Journal of Pharmacy and Pharmacology*, vol. 46 (1994): 1013–16.

22. K. Riehemann, B. Behnke, and K. Schulze Osthoff, "Plant Extracts from Stinging Nettle (*Urtica Dioica*), an Antirheumatic Remedy, Inhibit the Proinflammatory Transcription Factor NF-Kappab," *FEBS Letters*, vol. 442, no. 1 (1999): 89–94.

23. P. Mittman, "Randomized, Double-Blind Study of Freeze-Dried Urtica Dioica in the Treatment of Allergic Rhinitis," *Planta Medica.*, vol 56, no. 1 (1990): 44–47.

24. B. Obertreis, K. Giller, T. Teucher, B. Behnke, and H. Schmitz, "Anti-Inflammatory Effect of Urtica Dioica Folia Extract in Comparison to Caffeic Malic Acid Arzneimittelforschung," vol. 46, no.1 (1996): 52–56.

25. S. Chrubasik, W. Enderlein, R. Bauer, and W. Grabner, "Evidence for Antirheumatic Effectiveness of Herba Urtica Dioica in Acute Arthritis: A Pilot Study," *Phytomedicine*, vol. 4 (1997): 105–8.

26. Robert J. Peshek, *Balancing Body Chemistry with Nutrition* (NP: np, nd).

27. Y. Goso, Y. Ogata, K. Ishihara, and K. Hotta, "Effects of Traditional Herbal Medicine on Gastric Acid," *Biochemi Und Physiologie Der Pflanzen*, vol. 113C (1996): 17–21.

28. P. I. Reed and W. A. Davies, "Controlled Trial of a Carbenoxolone/Alginate Antacid Combination in Reflux Oesophagitis," *Current Medical Research and Opinion*, vol. 5 (1978): 637–44.

29. J. H. Liu, G. H. Chen, H. Z. Yeh, C. K. Huang, and S. K. Poon, "Enteric-Coated Peppermint-Oil Capsules in the Treatment of Irritable Bowel Syndrome: A Prospective, Randomized Trial," *Journal of Gastroenterology*, vol. 32, no. 6 (1997): 765–68.

30. J. Freise and S. Kohler, "Peppermint Oil-Caraway Oil Fixed Combination in Non-Ulcer Dyspepsia—Comparison of the Effects of Enteric Preparations," *Pharmazie*, vol. 54, no. 3 (1999): 210–15.

31. G. H. Micklefield, I. Greving, and B. May, "Effects of Peppermint Oil and Caraway Oil on Gastroduodenal Motility," *Phytotherapy Research*, vol. 14, no. 1 (2000): 20–23.

32. M. Blumenthal, et al., eds., *The Complete German Commission E Monographs.* (Austin, TX: Integrative Medicine Communications, 1998), p. 167.

33. P. J. Houghton, "The Scientific Basis for the Reputed Activity of Valerian," *The Journal of Pharmacy and Pharmacology*, vol. 51, no. 5 (1999): 505–12.

34. M. Bourin, T. Bougerol, B. Guitton, and E. Broutin, "A Combination of Plant Extracts in the Treatment of Outpatients with Adjustment Disorder with Anxious Mood: Controlled Study Versus Placebo," *Fundamental and Clinical Pharmacology*, vol. 11, no. 2 (1997): 127–32.

35. P. D. Leathwood, F. Chauffard, E. Heck, and R. Munoz-Box, "Aqueous Extract of Valerian Root (*Valeriana Officinalis L.*) Improves Sleep Quality in Man," *Pharmacology, Biochemistry and Behavior*, vol. 17, no. 1 (1982): 65–71.

36. *Alternative Medicine*, May 1994, p. 3.

37. Dan Bensky and Andrew Gamble, *Chinese Materia Medica* (Seattle, WA: Eastland Press, 1986).

38. M. Kubo, H. Matsuda, K. Tokuoka, S. Ma, and H. Shiomoto, "Anti-Inflammatory Activities of Methanolic Extract and Alkaloidal Components from Corydalis Tuber," *Biological and Phamaceutical Bulletin*, vol. 17, no. 2 (1994): 262–65.

39. L. Liu, G. Li, F. Zhu, L. Wang, and Y. Wang, "Comparison of Analgesic Effect Between Locally Vinegar-Processed Preparation of Fresh Rhizoma Corydalis and Traditionally Vinegar-Processed Rhizoma Corydalis," *Chung Kuo Chung Yao Tsa Chih*, vol. 15, no. 11 (1990): 666–67, 702.

40. F. Wei, S. Zou, A. Young, R. Dubner, and K. Ren, "Effects of Four Herbal Extracts on Adjuvant-Induced Inflammation and Hyperalgesia in Rats," *Journal of Alternative and Complementary Medicine*, vol. 5, no. 5 (1999): 429–36.

41. S. Mill, *Out of the Earth:* (London: Penguin, 1991), pp. 416–17.

42. M. Grieve, *A Modern Herbal* (New York: Dover, 1971), pp. 700–5.

43. David Hoffman, *The Complete Illustrated Holistic Herbal* (Rockport, MA: Element, 1996).

44. David Frawley and Vasant Lad, *The Yoga of Herbs* (Twin Lakes, WI: Lotus, 1986).

45. S. K. Jain and Robert A. DeFillips, *Medicinal Plants of India* (Algonac, MI: Reference Publications, 1991), p. 372.

46. K. M. Nadkarni, *Indian Materia Medica* (Bombay: Popular Prakashan, 1976), p. 863.

47. L. D. Kapoor, *The CRC Handbook of Ayurvedic Medicinal Plants* (Baton Rouge, LA: CRC Press, 1990), p. 249.

48. S. A. Phadke and S. D. Kulkarni, "Screening of In Vitro Antibacterial Activity of Terminalia Chebula, Eclapta Alba and Ocimum Sanctum," *Indian Journal of Medical Sciences*, vol. 43, no. 5 (1989): 113–17.

49. S. Godhwani, J. L. Godhwani, and D. S. Vyas, "Ocimum Sanctum—A Preliminary Study Evaluating Its Immunoregulatory Profile in Albino Rats," *Journal of Ethnopharmacology*, vol. 24, no. 2–3 (1988): 193–98.

50. R. Weiss, *Herbal Medicine* (Beaconsfield, England: Beaconsfield Publishers, 1988), pp. 228-29.

51. Personal communication.

52. R. Jovanovic, E. Congema, and H. T. Nguyen, "Antifungal Agents vs. Boric Acid for Treating Chronic Mycotic Vulvovaginitis," *Journal of Reproductive Medicine*, vol. 36, no. 8 (1991): 593–97.

53. K. K. Van Slyke, V. P. Michel, and M. F. Rein, "Treatment of Vulvovaginal Candidiasis with Boric Acid Powder," *American Journal of Obstetrics and Gynecology*, vol. 141, no. 2 (1981): 145–48.

54. Health Notes Online, http://www.gnc.com/health_notes/Supp/Boric_Acid.htm.

FOR MORE INFORMATION

Associations

American Association of Naturopathic Physicians
8201 Greensboro Drive
Suite 300
McLean, VA 22102
Phone: (703) 610-9037
Toll-free phone: (877) 969-2267
Fax: (703) 610-9005
Web site: www.naturopathic.org

American Association of Oriental Medicine
5530 Wisconsin Avenue
Suite 1210
Chevy Chase, MD 20815
Phone: (301) 941-1064
Toll-free phone: (888) 500-7999
Fax: (301) 986-9313
E-mail: hq@aaom.org
Web site: http://www.aaom.org

American Herbalists Guild
1931 Gaddis Road
Canton, GA 30115
Phone: (770) 751-6021

Fax: (770) 751-7472
E-mail: ahgoffice@earthlink.net
Web site: http://www.americanherbalist.com

American Holistic Medical Association
4101 Lake Boone Trail
Suite 201
Raleigh, NC 27607
Phone: (919) 787-5146
Web site: www.holisticmedicine.org

Green Farmacy Garden
James A. Duke, Ph.D., Botanist
8210 Murphy Road
Fulton, MD 20759
Phone: (301) 498-1175
E-mail: jimduke@comcast.net
Web site: www.ars-grin.gov/duke

Integrative Medical Arts Group
P.O. Box 671
Beaverton, OR 97075
Phone: (503) 526-1972
Web site: www.healthwwweb.com

Kundalini Yoga/3HO Foundation
Phone: (505) 753-4988
Toll-free phone: (888) 346-2420
Fax: (505) 753-1999
E-mail: yogainfo@3ho.org
Web site: www.3ho.org

National Center for Complementary and Alternative Medicine
National Institutes of Health
Bethesda, MD 20892
Web site: nccam.nih.gov

National Herbalists Association of Australia
33 Reserve Street
Annandale, NSW 2038

Phone: (02) 9560 7077
E-mail: nhaa@nhaa.org.au
Web site: www.nhaa.org.au

National Institute of Medical Herbalists (England)
56 Longbrook Street
Exeter EX4 6AH, UK
Phone: +44 (0) 1392 426022
Fax: +44 (0) 1392 498963
E-mail: nimh@ukexeter.freeserve.co.uk
Web site: http://www.nimh.org.uk

Recommended Reading

Aihara, Herman. *Acid and Alkaline*. George Oshawa Macrobiotic Foundation, 1986.

Baroody, Theodore A. *Alkalize or Die*. Holographic Health, 1991.

Bartram, Thomas. *Encyclopedia of Herbal Medicine*. Grace Publishers, 1995.

Beinfield, Harriet, and Efrem Korngold. *Between Heaven and Earth*. Ballantine Books, 1991.

Bensky, Dan, and Andrew Gamble. *Chinese Herbal Medicine: Materia Medica*. Eastland Press, 1993.

Blumenthal et al. *The Complete German Commission E Monographs*. Integrative Medicine Communications, 1998.

Brown, Susan E. *Better Bones, Better Body: A Comprehensive Self-Help Program for Preventing, Halting and Overcoming Osteoporosis*. Keats, 1996.

Brown, Susan E. *Better Bones, Better Body: Beyond Estrogen and Calcium*. Contemporary Books, 2000.

Erasmus, Udo. *Fats That Heal, Fats That Kill*. Alive Books, 1986.

Flaws, Bob. *The Book of Jook: Chinese Medicinal Porridges*. Blue Poppy Press, 1995.

Flaws, Bob. *My Sister the Moon: The Diagnosis and Treatment of Menstrual Diseases by Traditional Chinese Medicine*. Blue Poppy Press, 1992.

Frawley, David. *Ayurvedic Healing*. Passage Press, 1989.

Gaby, Alan. *Preventing and Reversing Osteoporosis: What You Can Do About Bone Loss*. Prima, 1995.

Griggs, Barbara. *Green Pharmacy*. Healing Arts Press, 1997.

Haller, John S. *Kindly Medicine*. Kent State University Press, 1997.

Haller, John S. *Medical Protestants*. Southern Illinois University Press, 1994.

Holmes, Peter. *The Energetics of Western Herbs*. Snow Lotus Press, 1997.

Lad, Vasant. *Ayurveda: The Science of Self-Healing*. Lotus Press, 1984.

Lad, Vasant, and David Frawley. *Yoga of Herbs*. Lotus Press, 1986.

Landis, Robyn, and Karta Purkh Singh Khalsa. *Herbal Defense*. Warner Books, 1997.

Lininger, Skye et al. *The Natural Pharmacy*. Prima, 1998.

Mills, Simon, and Kerry Bone. *Principles and Practice of Phytotherapy*. Churchill Livingstone, 2000.

Svoboda, Robert E. *Ayurveda: Life, Health and Longevity*. Arkana, 1992.

Tierra, Lesley. *Healing with Chinese Herbs*. The Crossing Press, 1997.

Tierra, Lesley. *The Herbs of Life*. The Crossing Press, 1992.

Tierra, Michael. *Planetary Herbology*. Lotus Press, 1988.

Tierra, Michael, and Lesley Tierra. *Chinese-Planetary Herbal Diagnosis: A Primer*. Tierra, 1988.

Tierra, Michael, and Lesley Tierra. *Chinese Traditional Herbal Medicine*. Lotus Press, 1998.

Tillotson, Alan. *The One Earth Herbal Sourcebook*. Twin Streams, 2001.

Wiley, Rudolf A. *BioBalance*. Essential Science Publishing, 1989.

BIBLIOGRAPHY

Aihara, Herman. *Acid and Alkaline*. Oroville, CA: George Oshawa Macrobiotic Foundation, 1986.

Baker, Sidney MacDonald. *Detoxification and Healing*. New Canaan, CT: Keats, 1997.

Baroody, Theodore A. *Alkalize or Die*. Waynesville, NC: Holographic Health, 1991.

Bartram, Thomas. *Encyclopedia of Herbal Medicine*. Christchurch, Dorset, England: Grace Publishers, 1995.

Beinfield, Harriet, and Efrem Korngold. *Between Heaven and Earth*. New York: Ballantine Books, 1991.

Bensky, Dan, and Andrew Gamble. *Chinese Herbal Medicine: Materia Medica*. Seattle, WA: Eastland Press, 1993.

Blumenthal, M. et al., Eds. *The Complete German Commission E Monographs*. Austin, TX: Integrative Medicine Communications, 1998.

Brown, Susan E. *Better Bones, Better Body: A Comprehensive Self-Help Program for Preventing, Halting and Overcoming Osteoporosis*. New Canaan, CT: Keats, 1996.

Brown, Susan E. *Better Bones, Better Body: Beyond Estrogen and Calcium*. New York: Contemporary Books, 2000.

Erasmus, Udo. *Fats That Heal, Fats That Kill*. Burnaby, BC, Canada: Alive Books, 1986.

Flaws, Bob. *The Book of Jook: Chinese Medicinal Porridges*. Boulder, CO: Blue Poppy Press, 1995.

Flaws, Bob. *My Sister the Moon: The Diagnosis and Treatment of Menstrual*

Diseases by Traditional Chinese Medicine. Boulder, CO: Blue Poppy Press, 1992.

Frawley, David. *Ayurvedic Healing*. Salt Lake City, UT: Passage Press, 1989.

Gaby, Alan. *Preventing and Reversing Osteoporosis: What You Can Do About Bone Loss*. Rocklin, CA: Prima, 1995.

Gaeddert, Andrew. *Chinese Herbs in the Western Clinic*. Berkeley, CA: North Atlantic Books, 1998.

Griggs, Barbara. *Green Pharmacy*. Rochester, VT: Healing Arts Press, 1997.

Haller, John S. *Kindly Medicine*. Kent, OH: Kent State University Press, 1997.

Haller, John S. *Medical Protestants*. Carbondale: Southern Illinois University Press, 1994.

Holmes, Peter. *Energetics of Western Herbs*. Boulder, CO: Snow Lotus Press, 1997.

Hsu, Hong-Yen and Peacher. *Chinese Herbal Medicine and Therapy*. Long Beach, CA: Oriental Healing Arts Institute, 1994.

Kaptchuk, Ted. *The Web That Has No Weaver*. New York: Contemporary Books, 2000.

Krohn, Jacqueline, and Frances Taylor. *Natural Detoxification*. Berkeley, CA: Hartley & Marks, 2000.

Lad, Vasant. *Ayurveda: The Science of Self-Healing*. Wilmot, WI: Lotus, 1984.

Lad, Vasant, and David Frawley. *The Yoga of Herbs*. Santa Fe, NM: Lotus, 1986.

Landis, Robyn, and Karta Purkh Singh Khalsa. *Herbal Defense*. New York: Warner Books, 1997.

Lininger, Skye et al. *The Natural Pharmacy*. Rocklin, CA: Prima, 1998.

Mills, Simon, and Kerry Bone. *Principles and Practice of Phytotherapy*. London: Churchill Livingstone, 2000.

Pang, T. Y. *Chinese Herbal*. Honolulu, HI: Tai Chi School of Philosophy and Art, 1982.

Reid, Daniel. *Chinese Herbal Medicine*. Boston: Shambala Publications, 1986.

Reid, Daniel. *Complete Book of Chinese Health and Healing*. Boston: Shambala Publications, 1995.

Svoboda, Robert E. *Ayurveda: Life, Health and Longevity*. London: Arkana, 1992.

Teeguarden, Ron. *Chinese Tonic Herbs*. Tokyo: Japan Publications, 1985.

Tierra, Lesley. *Healing with Chinese Herbs*. Berkeley, CA: The Crossing Press, 1997.

Tierra, Lesley. *The Herbs of Life*. Berkeley, CA: The Crossing Press, 1992.

Tierra, Michael. *Planetary Herbology*. Santa Fe, NM: Lotus Press, 1988.

Tierra, Michael, and Lesley Tierra. *Chinese-Planetary Herbal Diagnosis: A Primer*. Np: Tierra, 1988.

Tierra, Michael, and Lesley Tierra. *Chinese Traditional Herbal Medicine*. Santa Fe, NM: Lotus Press, 1998.

Tillotson Alan. *The One Earth Herbal Sourcebook*. New York: Twin Streams, 2001.

Vokovic, Laurel. *14-Day Herbal Cleansing*. Upper Saddle River, NJ: Prentice-Hall, 1998.

Wiley, Rudolf A. *BioBalance*. Hurricane, UT: Essential Science Publishing, Utah, 1989.

RESOURCE LIST

Natural Medicine Resources

Aika Boost
Electrolyte Dietary Supplement
(714) 248-7512/(800) 861-0513

Ancient Healing Ways
Ayurvedic Herbs and Yoga Supplies
(877) 753-5351
www.a-healing.com

Dr. Susan E. Brown
Better Bones-Better Body® pH Test Kit
(315) 432-9231
www.betterbones.com/products.htm

Dharma Singh Khalsa, MD (best-selling author)
info@drdharma.com
(520) 749-8374
www.drdharma.com

Dr. Susan Lark Products
(888) 314-LARK
E-mail: dpics@drlark.com
www.drlark.com

Metabolic Testing

Harold J. Kristal DDS
Phone: (800) 722-0646
E-mail: hkristal@bloodph.com
www.bloodph.com

Great Smokies Diagnostic Laboratory
800-522-4762
www.gsdl.com

Health Equations
Health equation blood test
Tel. (802) 365-9213
Fax (802) 365-9218
www.healthequation.com

Nutri-Spec
Urine and saliva testing to determine metabolic imbalances
(800) 736-4320
www.nutri-spec.net

Homecure, Inc.
pH Charts, Equipment and Books
(480) 443-3373
(800) 559-2873

Nutritional Supplements and Herbal Products

The list below contains companies whose product lines can be relied upon for both quality and reliability. For further detailed information on any company listed, either call the toll-free telephone number or check its website. Most of the products can be found at your local health food store or obtained through your physician.

American Herbal Products Association
http://www.ahpa.org/

Carotec, Inc.
800-522-4279
www.carotec.com

Gaia Herbs
800-831-7780
www.gaiaherbs.com

Garden of Life
800-622-8986
www.gardenoflifeusa.com or www.gardenoflife.com

Healthy Origins
888-228-6650
www.healthyorigins.com

Herbalist and Alchemist
http://www.herbalist-alchemist.com/

Jarrow Formulas
800-726-0886
www.Jarrow.com

J.R. Carlson Laboratories, Inc.
888-234-5656
www.carlsonlabs.com

Longevity Plus
800-580-PLUS (7587)
www.longevityplus.net

Longevity Science
800-933-9440
www.longevity-science.net

Metagenics
http://www.metagenics.com/

Planetary Formulas
800-606-6226
www.planetaryformulas.com

Source Naturals Inc.
800-815-2333
www.sourcenaturals.com

Thorne Research
800-228-1966
www.thorne.com

Vitamin Research Products
800-877-2447
www.vrp.com

Environmental Products

N.E.E.D.S.
800-634-1380
www.needs.com
This is a total resource for every type of environmental product that is on the market today. They stock air cleaners for house and car and have special air cleaners available for multiple chemical sensitivities. They also stock specific airborne chemical product filters. Filters for airborne mold, toxins and biological problems are also available. They carry the Doulton Water Filter, shower filters and many other environmental products.

Organic Foods, Teas and Oils

Bragg Live Foods
Bragg's Aminos
Bragg's Organic Apple Cider Vinegar
(800) 446-1990
www.bragg.com

Flaxseeds

Living Tree Community Foods
800-260-5534
www.livingtreecommunity.com
Organic Golden Flax
Golden flaxseeds are larger and softer than the dark brown flaxseeds. They have a mild nutty flavor that is really delicious mixed in food. It is also a known source of potassium, magnesium, and boron.

Omega Nutrition
800-661-3529
www.omeganutrition.com

The Grain and Salt Society
Celtic Sea Salt
(800) 867-7258
www.celticseasalt.com

Tree of Life
www.treeoflife.com
Many health food stores are supplied by a company known as Tree of Life, a distributor of high quality natural foods at moderate prices. Among the many products they carry are frozen organic vegetables, organic fruits, organic extra virgin olive oil, organic tomato sauce products, and many others.

Vitamin Research Products
Flax Seed
800-877-2447
www.vrp.com
Dakota Flax Gold. These tiny golden seeds have a rich nutty flavor. Available in seed form.

OLIVE OIL

Living Tree Community Foods
(800) 260-5534
www.livingtreecommunity.com
Living Tree has a raw organic olive oil that is not pressed. It's centrifuged at 75 degrees Fahrenheit, room temperature.

RICE BRAN SYRUP

Bernard Jensen International
(888) 743-1790
www.bernardjensen.org

POULTRY

Sheltons Poultry, Inc.
(800) 541-1833
www.sheltons.com
Free-range chickens and turkeys with no added antibiotics. The taste quality of these natural products is far superior to products that are laced with all sorts of additives and hormones. Available in natural food stores.

SEAFOOD (WILD CAUGHT)

Seafood Direct
(800) 732-1836
www.buyseafooddirect.com
A wonderful source for non-farmed fish including salmon, tuna, and others.

SWEETENERS

Omega Nutrition
(800) 661-3529
www.omegahealthstore.com
A selection of stevia products in powdered form, liquid form, and also packet form.

Vitamin Research Products
(800) 877-2447
www.vrp.com

Unique Sweet
(Xylitol Crystals)
A unique sweetener in powdered form. Also available in a variety of Xylitol gums.

Wisdom of the Ancients
(800) 899-9908
www.wisdomherbs.com
Natural sweetener made from whole leaf stevia (*Stevia rebaudiana Bertoni*) 6:1 concentrated extract. Available in concentrated tablets, liq-

uid, and as a tea. Hundreds of scientific studies have been conducted on stevia's effectiveness as a nutritional addition to the diet.

TEA

Maitake Products, Inc.
(800) 747-7418
www.maitake.com
Maigreen™ Tea
Contains organically grown maitake mushroom and premier Japanese green tea (matcha) leaves. Low in caffeine. Available in tea bags.

Rishi Tea
(866) 747-4483 (866-RISHI TEA)
www.rishi-tea.com
Rishi offers more than two dozen certified organic teas, including ten green tea varietals. While the positive health benefits of regular consumption of green tea are now well documented, this company sells only high quality loose tea including Rooibos Tea, Pu-erh Tea, White Tea, and others.

Triple Leaf Tea, Inc.
(800) 552-7448
www.tripleleaf-tea.com
Effective authentic, traditional Chinese green, naturally decaffeinated green, medicinal and diet teas, made with authentic Chinese herbs and traditional herbal formulas, packaged in convenient tea bag form. All teas are GMO-free. Triple Leaf's Decaf Green Tea and Decaf Green Tea blends uses a natural solvent-free carbon dioxide decaffeination process. They also carry Decaf Green Tea with Ginseng, Ginko and Decaf Green Tea, American Ginseng Herbal Tea, Ginger Root Tea and Detox Tea.

WATER

Mountain Valley Spring Water
(800) 643-1501
www.mountainvalleyspring.com
This water company has been bottling and distributing their pure

spring water since 1871. They are one of the few bottled water companies that still offer some of their products in glass.

Penta™ Purified Drinking Water
(800) 531-5088
www.hydrateforlife.com
This company uses a system of purifying their water that has less dissolved solvents than either distilled or reverse osmosis purified water.

INDEX